Communications
in Computer and Information Science   **556**

Commenced Publication in 2007
Founding and Former Series Editors:
Alfredo Cuzzocrea, Dominik Ślęzak, and Xiaokang Yang

More information about this series at http://www.springer.com/series/7899

Jan Cabri · João Barreiros
Pedro Pezarat-Correia (Eds.)

Sports Science Research and Technology Support

Second International Congress, icSPORTS 2014
Rome, Italy, October 24–26, 2014
Revised Selected Papers

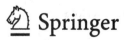 Springer

Editors
Jan Cabri
Norwegian School of Sport Sciences
Oslo
Norway

Pedro Pezarat-Correia
Universidade de Lisboa
Cruz Quebrada
Portugal

João Barreiros
Universidade de Lisboa
Cruz Quebrada
Portugal

ISSN 1865-0929   ISSN 1865-0937 (electronic)
Communications in Computer and Information Science
ISBN 978-3-319-25248-3   ISBN 978-3-319-25249-0 (eBook)
DOI 10.1007/978-3-319-25249-0

Library of Congress Control Number: 2015950455

Springer Cham Heidelberg New York Dordrecht London

Printed on acid-free paper

Springer International Publishing AG Switzerland is part of Springer Science+Business Media
(www.springer.com)

Preface

The present book includes extended and revised versions of a set of selected papers from the Second International Congress on Sport Sciences Research and Technology Support (icSPORTS 2014), held in Rome, Italy, during October 24–26, 2014.

The purpose of the International Congress on Sport Sciences Research and Technology Support is to bring together researchers and practitioners in order to exchange ideas and developed synergies highlighting the benefits of any kind of technology for sports, either in general or regarding a particular case of application.

icSPORTS 2014 was sponsored by the Institute for Systems and Technologies of Information, Control and Communication (INSTICC) and had the institutional sponsorship of Universidade de Lisboa (Faculdade de Motricidade Humana), the Olympic Committee of Portugal, and the Norwegian School of Sport Sciences. It was held in cooperation with the European College of Sport Science (ECSS); European College of Sports and Exercise Physicians (ECOSEP); International Association of Computer Science in Sport (IACSS); Società Italiana delle Scienze Motorie e Sportive; European Federation of Sport Psychology; Società Italiana di Anatomia; IASK - International Association of Sport Kinetics; European Association for Sport Management. icSPORTS 2014 also had as R&D group partners the following projects: BLIND-TRACK (guiding system for visually impaired for individual running on the track) and REPOPA (research into policy to enhance physical activity).

The congress received 131 paper submissions from 37 countries in all continents. To evaluate each submission, a double-blind paper review was performed by the Program Committee. After a stringent selection process, 14 papers were published and presented as full papers, i.e., completed work (30' oral presentation), leading to a "full-paper" acceptance ratio of about 11.5 %, which shows the intention of preserving a high-quality forum for the next editions of this congress.

icSPORTS's program included panels and four invited talks delivered by internationally distinguished speakers, namely: Luis Paulo Reis (University of Minho, Portugal), Peter Federolf (Norwegian University for Science and Technology, Norway), Antoine Nordez (University of Nantes, France), and Hermano Igo Krebs (Massachusetts Institute of Technology, USA).

We would like to thank the authors, whose research and development efforts are recorded here for future generations.

April 2015

Jan Cabri
João Barreiros
Pedro Pezarat-Correia
Laura Capranica

Organization

Congress Chair

Jan Cabri   Norwegian School of Sport Sciences, Norway

Program Co-chairs

João Barreiros   Faculdade de Motricidade Humana/Universidade de Lisboa, Portugal

Pedro Pezarat-Correia   Faculdade de Motricidade Humana/Universidade de Lisboa, Portugal

Local Chair

Laura Capranica   Università degli Studi di Roma "Foro Italico", Italy

Organizing Committee

Helder Coelhas	INSTICC, Portugal
Lucia Gomes	INSTICC, Portugal
Ana Guerreiro	INSTICC, Portugal
André Lista	INSTICC, Portugal
Andreia Moita	INSTICC, Portugal
Vitor Pedrosa	INSTICC, Portugal
Cláudia Pinto	INSTICC, Portugal
João Ribeiro	INSTICC, Portugal
Susana Ribeiro	INSTICC, Portugal
Sara Santiago	INSTICC, Portugal
Mara Silva	INSTICC, Portugal
José Varela	INSTICC, Portugal
Pedro Varela	INSTICC, Portugal

Program Committee

María Ángeles Pérez Ansón	University of Zaragoza, Spain
Duarte Araújo	Universidade de Lisboa, Portugal
Arnold Baca	University of Vienna, Austria
Bill Baltzopoulos	Brunel University, UK
José Angelo Barela	Universidade Cruzeiro do Sul, Brazil
Karl-Peter Benedetto	Landeskrankenhaus Feldkirch, Austria
Rodrigo Rico Bini	Universidade Federal do Rio Grande do Sul, Brazil

Andrew Kilding	Auckland University of Technology, New Zealand
Mark King	Loughborough University, UK
Andrey Koptyug	Mid Sweden University, Sweden
Nicola Lai	Case Western Reserve University, USA
Anthony Leicht	James Cook University, Australia
Silvio Lorenzetti	Institute for Biomechanics, ETH Zurich, Switzerland
Sean Maw	Mount Royal University, Canada
Melitta McNarry	Swansea University, UK
Chris Mills	University of Portsmouth, UK
Fabio Nakamura	Universidade Estadual de Londrina, Brazil
Mitsuo Ochi	Hiroshima University, Japan
I. Mark Olfert	West Virginia University, USA
Raul A.N.S. Oliveira	Universidade de Lisboa, Portugal
Matthew Pain	Loughborough University, UK
António Labisa Palmeira	Universidade Lusófona de Humanidades e Tecnologias, Portugal
Evangelos Pappas	University of Sydney, Australia
Pedro Passos	Universidade de Lisboa, Portugal
Carl Payton	Manchester Metropolitan University, UK
José Miguel Dias Pereira	Escola Superior de Tecnologia de Setúbal, Portugal
Noel Perkins	University of Michigan, USA
Alessandro Pezzoli	DIST - Politecnico di Torino and Università di Torino, Italy
David Rowlands	Griffith University, Australia
Scott Sailor	California State University, Fresno, USA
Alison Sheets	Nike Sports Research Lab, USA
Luís Silva	Universidade Lusiada, Portugal
James S. Skinner	Indiana University, USA
Christos Spitas	Delft University of Technology, The Netherlands
Kazumoto Tanaka	Kinki University, Japan
Normand Teasdale	Laval University, Canada
David Thiel	Griffith University, Australia
Rui Torres	North Polytechnic Institute of Health, Paredes, Portugal
Herbert Ugrinowitsch	Universidade Federal de Minas Gerais, Brazil
Kirsti Uusi-Rasi	UKK Institute for Health Promotion Research, Finland
Benedicte Vanwanseele	KU Leuven, Belgium
J. Paulo Vilas-Boas	Universidade do Porto, Portugal
Eric Wallace	University of Ulster, UK
Hans Weghorn	BW Cooperative State University Stuttgart, Germany
Edward Winter	Sheffield Hallam University, UK
Yanxin Zhang	The University of Auckland, New Zealand

Additional Reviewer

| Sarah Dennis | University of Sydney, Australia |

Invited Speakers

Luis Paulo Reis	University of Minho, Portugal
Peter Federolf	Norwegian University for Science and Technology, Norway
Antoine Nordez	University of Nantes, France
Hermano Igo Krebs	Massachusetts Institute of Technology, USA

Contents

Development of Skill Scoring System for Ski and Snowboard

Shinichi Yamagiwa[1][✉], Hiroyuki Ohshima[1], and Kazuki Shirakawa[2]

[1] Faculty of Engineering, Information and Systems, University of Tsukuba,
Tsukuba, Japan
{yamagiwa,ohshima}@cs.tsukuba.ac.jp
http://www.cs.tsukuba.ac.jp/~yamagiwa/
[2] Exercise Physiology, Health Education, Graduate School of Education,
Hokkaido University, Sapporo, Japan
kazuki.shirakawa@edu.hokudai.ac.jp

Abstract. Observation of dynamic posture during sports activity is one of the most important factors to give absolute evaluation to the player's performance. The sports like the figure skating and the skiing have difficulty in evaluation of skill because the evaluation depends mostly on the observation from the third person. The training method for such sports inevitably needs feedback comments from the experts. However, it is hard for all players of the sports to receive such expensive feedbacks at any time when they need. In order to overcome the inconvenience to perform self-training without the third experts, this paper focuses on development of a training system using smartphone device that gives a clear guide for body balance control in the skier and the snowboarder. The system gives scores and comments for the ski's parallel turn. The system automatically scores skill for body balance control regarding three aspects: the tempo at turns of body balance movements between the right and the left in the skiing, the distribution of body balance, and the angle between the snow slope and the body of the skier. This paper also performs a preliminary evaluation of the system in the case of snowboard. The system brings a new method to know the skills of body balance control in skiing and snowboarding from the absolute data measured by sensor devices.

Keywords: Ski · Snowboard · Skill scoring · Gamification · Trainig system

1 Introduction

The skill level of any sports activity relates to the appearance of performance. If a player performs well, the dynamic posture of his performance should be elegant. However, the player is not able to observe himself from multiple aspects, only observation by the third person can bring the judge of the skill level. In some sports, the judge of the skill level is brought by the observation. For example, in figure skating, the player is evaluated by judges according to the appearance

© Springer International Publishing Switzerland 2015
J. Cabri et al. (Eds.): icSPORTS 2014, CCIS 556, pp. 1–15, 2015.
DOI: 10.1007/978-3-319-25249-0_1

of the performance. Moreover, skiing is one of the major sports that evaluates appearance during the performance. The qualification tests mainly in Japan, Canada and New Zealand perform examinations by checking the level of the ski skill from observation of the appearance during the performance [3]. One of the important performance skills in ski is a smooth parallel turn in a gentle snow slope. A major training method for the parallel turn is to hear comments from high skill trainers who have been qualified by the trainer license test, or to check movies during gliding in the snow slope and to get the comments from the high skill skiers. Thus, it is impossible to train the parallel turn by the skier himself without any objective comments.

Regarding the ski's parallel turn, there exist several engineering analysis of the dynamic posture. For example, a ski robot [5] and a simulation-based quantitative approach [1] were performed. These investigated modeling methods of the dynamic posture of skiing. However, these are not targeted to use it for training the skill. Moreover, another modeling method for the dynamic posture applying accelerometer, magnetic sensor and GPS was also proposed by [2]. Including this method, all those advanced researches did not discuss by what the parallel turn becomes elegance. Considering the qualification test explained above, the skiers aim to acquire the skill that maintains elegant and dynamic posture during the parallel turns.

This paper will propose a system called *ski trainer* that provides scoring methods for the performance of ski's parallel turn and also provides how elegance the performance is. How elegant is evaluated by the dynamic posture of skier regarding the tempo, the symmetry and the distribution of body balance. The score is calculated based on data from the actual accelerometer, and then, the system feedbacks advices for directing the next step of the training.

In the next section, this paper describes the backgrounds and definitions regarding the skill acquisition process of skiing. Section 3 will propose the ski trainer system discussing the methods to score the dynamic posture. Section 4 will show the evaluation of the system regarding the effects and the validity of the system. Finally we will conclude the paper and mention the future plans.

2 Backgrounds and Definitions

2.1 Training Methods Using Advanced Devices in Sports

It is a very hard process for an athlete to evaluate self-performance of sports by giving scores without guide for the ideal target performance. It is mandatory for a coach or a trainer or an expert player to give comments to the player from the appearance of the dynamic posture. However, the target direction to change the form or the posture should be presented by some absolute standard. The best way is to apply standardized values measured by sensors as the guide to cause the ideal dynamic posture.

Advanced technologies in these days implement internet-based communities using small sensor technologies (so called, MEMS) equipped in such as a smartphone. The mobile devices include accelerometer, gyro sensors and GPS. For example, Otsuka et al. implemented a social network system (SNS) that provides a community to encourage runners of jogging by the participants in the system [4]. Using position information from GPS of a runner, the system shows an ideal and the actual speed of the runner. Nike+ (http://nikeplus. nike.com/), which is available in iPhone in these days, is also the similar system that returns the information of the positions during jogging. Adidas' micoach (http://micoach.adidas.com/) is also another system to guide physical threshold of runner's body. It uses heart beat information to guide physical availability of the runner. However, these system shows only how much wrong or how much different from the ideal target values. Therefore the users of the systems can not know how to improve the skill using the information from the systems.

2.2   Training Methods and Qualification for Skiing

In this paper we focus on skiing. There is a skill qualification in Japan, so called *badge test* organized by SAJ (Ski Association of Japan) (http://www.ski-japan. or.jp/). To pass the qualification examination, skiers need to join in a training course and receive comments from the expert trainers. The qualification is mainly decided by the appearance of the performance. The decision of the qualification depends on observations by a few expert trainers during the examination. Therefore, it is hard to standardize the level of the qualification among different ski resorts or different snow slopes.

In Canada and New Zealand, there are the similar qualification licensing examinations organized by Nonstop (http://www.nonstopsnow.com/). This also causes the same problem as the one of Japan mentioned above.

The training to get good skill for passing the qualification test is mainly to watch the video or to receive comments from the experts. However, it is hard for all skiers to get such guides from experts. Therefore, it is important to implement a system that provides training directions for skiers using absolute body's movement data measured by sensors.

2.3   Discussion

As mentioned above, it is hard for skier by himself to acquire the higher level skill without observing appearance of his performance. Therefore, sensor data brings possibility to train him without any comments from the experts. Such as the systems for jogging discussed above, the similar system is needed for skiing. However, sensor grabs not only the dynamic posture to the skier, but the next step for getting higher skill should be shown by the system. If not, the skier needs the experts' comments again to understand the data from sensors.

This paper will show development of a scoring system called *Ski Trainer* based on data analysis using the skills of experts. Additionally the system will give advices to the user skier to acquire the higher skill. The system applies the sensors to acquire the motions of skier and calculates the skill level. Then the system will give the comments to the skier.

We expect the *gamification* effect according to the feedback information from the ski trainer system. The skier will try to get higher scores from the system. It promotes the encouragement for the skier to reach higher skill level by showing the score of the current skill and also by giving advices to jump up to the next skill level.

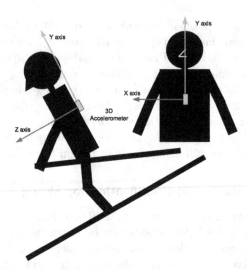

Fig. 1. The measurement axis of accelerometer piggybacked by skier.

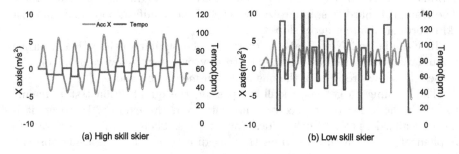

Fig. 2. A tempo graph example.

3 Ski Trainer System

3.1 Methods for Scoring

We use an accelerometer to measure performance of skier. We defined the axes of the sensor as shown in Fig. 1. We have used data from the accelerometer with three dimensional axis focusing on the three aspects as described below. Here we use 200 Hz sampling data for the analysis.

1. Tempo
   When a skier glides in a static tempo, the skier has ability to adapt himself to any snow surface. This means his skill is high if he can follow the tempo. According to this technical aspect, we apply tempo to evaluate the skier's skill. When we plot the X axis of the accelerometer values to the vertical axis of a graph as shown in Fig. 2, the tempo is calculated by measuring the time distances of crossing points with the horizontal axis of the origin (i.e. X value

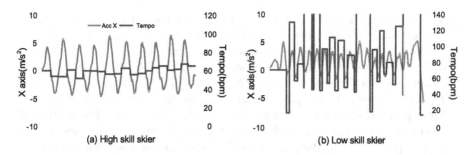

Fig. 3. Comparison of tempo between (a) a high skill skier (the upper) and (b) a low skill one (the lower).

of accelerometer becomes zero). Let us consider the i-th crossing point $t(i)$ sec. The tempo $T(i)$ is calculated by $(t(i+1) - t(i)) \times 60$ bpm. Here, we apply a threshold condition $T(i) = T + T_H$ when $|T(i) - T| > T_H$ and $T_H \leq T$. This threshold is needed for limiting to the domain of $T(i)$ less than $T + T_H$ because the skier would mistake to turn in a much earlier timing than the target timing. The distribution of the tempo is defined by;

$$\rho = \sqrt{\frac{\sum_{i=0}^{N-1}\{(T(i) - T)^2\}}{N}} \tag{1}$$

$$M = (\frac{\rho}{T} \times 100) \tag{2}$$

where $0 < i < N$ and T is the target tempo decided by the skier. The score is calculated by $100 - M$. Here, we use $T_H = T$.

Figure 3 shows an example of calculation of $T(i)$ used in the equation above. The upper waves than the horizontal axis of origin show the left side turns. Besides, the lower waves show the right side turns. Figure 3 illustrates the comparison of the tempo graph between a high and a low skill skiers. Figure 3(a) shows the one of a high skill skier with the badge test qualification. Figure 3(b) shows the tempo graph of a low skill skier. Here, each skier defines the target tempo as a suitable turn timings at which he performs parallel turns easily. The high skill skier follows the stable tempo of 60 bpm. However, another skier does not follow the target tempo, for which he targets to the one of 70 bpm. Thus, the tempo is one of the important aspects to decide the skill of skier. Using the distribution calculated by the Eq. (1), we can represent the score to inform the skier's skill. This means that the skier can know the level with a numerical and absolute value and they can understand what the main target to accomplish is. According to the movement data analysis, the skier will try to train the skill to glide any slope at a concrete and stable tempo.

2. Symmetry

A good balance between the right and the left side during gliding with parallel turn is mandatory for maintaining a good form of skiing. The balance is evaluated by two aspects. One is the ratio of body balance movement between the right and the left sides. We call this the *balance ratio*. Another is the angles of body against the snow slope during turns. We call this the *balance angle*. These are analyzed by the accelerometer's X-Y data mapped to a scatter diagram. Figure 4(a) shows the scatter diagram. The raw data from the accelerometer during parallel turn shapes like a reversed V character. The top of the diagram of Y axis is 9.8 m/s^2, which is 1G. The bottom of it becomes 2G because there does not exist any force from the head to the snow slope more than the gravity as illustrated in Fig. 4(a). When we move data to Y direction for 1G (Step 1 in Fig. 4(a)) and replace the sign of each Y value of the point (Step 2 in Fig. 4(a)), it becomes like a V character such as Fig. 4(b). Using this diagram, we decide the scores for the balance ratio and the balance angle. We call this diagram the *symmetry diagram* in this paper.

Regarding the balance ratio, we count the numbers of points in the diagram separating the right and the left side of the Y axis. If a side against Y axis has a larger number of points, the body balance causes an inclination to the side. If the both sides have the same number of points, it keeps ideal symmetry balance for the parallel turn that obtains well balance between the right and the left sides of the body. Thus, we score the balance ratio using the equation below;

$$100 - \frac{|L_y - R_y|}{L_y + R_y} \times 100 \tag{3}$$

where L_y is the number of points in the left side and R_y is the one of the right side against Y axis in the diagram.

On the other hand, the balance angle is calculated by processing an approximated line from the origin of the symmetry diagram of Fig. 4(b). How to calculate the line is shown in the Appendix section. For example, it shows the lines from the origin of the diagram to the left and the right sides against Y axis as depicted in Fig. 4(b). When the angles of those lines are respectively a_L and a_R, we calculate the score using the equations below;

$$100 - 100 \times (\frac{|a_L|}{|a_R|} - 1), |a_L| \geq |a_R| \tag{4}$$

$$100 - 100 \times (\frac{|a_R|}{|a_L|} - 1), |a_L| < |a_R| \tag{5}$$

If this ratio is more than 100 or less than 50, the score is 0 because it means that the body balance between the right and the left sides differs widely.

3. Dynamicity

We have experimented with six participants to measure the maximum acceleration to the left and the right side of the body balance. Figure 5(a) shows the symmetry diagram with four time trials of parallel turns performed by a high skill skier. It does not become more than 2G (9.8 $m/s^2 \times 2 = 19.6\ m/s^2$) to the right and the left side. On the other hand, as a comparison, the case of the low skill skier shows that the domain of data between the right and the left sides becomes small as depicted in Fig. 5(b). In this case, the appearance of the parallel turns becomes compact and is not elegant. When the acceleration to both sides is maintained largely, the appearance of the parallel

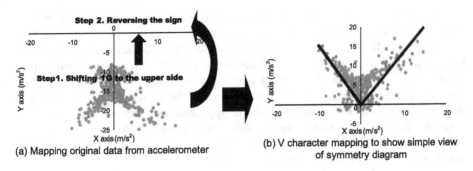

Fig. 4. Scatter diagram of a V character mapping X-Y axis of accelerometer data. When we move the data for 1G from the original and reverse the sign of the data regarding Y direction, the shape becomes like a V character.

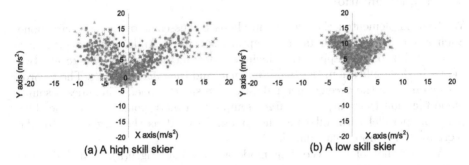

Fig. 5. Symmetry diagrams of (a) a high skill and (b) a low skill skiers. The force to the right and the left sides never become more than 2G. The data domain in the case of low skill skier becomes small.

turn seems elegant because the angle of the body becomes keen against snow slope. This means that the skier is able to control widely his body balance during the parallel turns. Therefore, we decide the score for the dynamicity to provide a higher score when a larger acceleration is observed from data of the accelerometer using the equation below;

$$((\frac{L_{max} + R_{max}}{2})/19.6) \times 100 \tag{6}$$

where the maximum acceleration to the left and the right are L_{max} and R_{max} respectively. This equation calculates an average among L_{max} and R_{max}, and the ratio is calculated by dividing 2G.

Applying the tempo, the symmetry and the dynamicity to the scoring methods, we can evaluate the skier's skill of his parallel turn technique as mentioned above. The tempo shows the ability of the skier if he can adapt himself to the snow surface. The symmetry gives advice to correct skier's turn to obtain it beautiful. The dynamicity brings a factor if he can perform elegant parallel turn.

The scoring methods bring a new feature for the training system, which extends the system to output messages used as advices to the skier. We define the messages regarding the scores for the tempo, the symmetry and the dynamicity. When the score of tempo is more than 80, it outputs a message "gliding in a good tempo". If it is less than 40, it outputs "follow the target tempo". When the score of balance angle is 0, it shows a message "inclination is too significant" to the right or the left according to the approximation line in the symmetry diagram. If it is 50 or more, the message "the balance is good" is outputted. When the score of dynamicity is more than 70, it outputs "elegant gliding". If not, it shows "use more side edges to line curves".

Using these three scoring methods and messaging output rules, we implement a system for ski's parallel turn called *Ski Trainer*.

3.2   Implementation

We have implemented the scoring methods discussed above in a smartphone application. The screenshots of the application in an Android smartphone are shown in Fig. 6. The application includes the functions below. There are two modes in the application: the *recording mode* and the *analysis mode*. The recording mode saves the accelerometer data to the smartphone. It includes a sound guide function that outputs a target tempo by a metronome sound. The skier performs parallel turn following the sound. Using it as the target tempo, the score for the tempo is calculated.

A screenshot of the recording mode is shown in Fig. 6(a). It includes the accelerometer data and the gyroscope data measured by the sensors equipped in the smartphone. The STBY button starts to record the motion data and saves it in a CSV file stored in the smartphone.

The analysis mode has three steps to show the scores. The first step is to select the interval of the parallel turns as shown in Fig. 6(b). This is done by a touch and a drag operation to select the duration of the parallel turns. The ski trainer application has a comparing function among several performances at a time. Therefore, the second step selects data sets to evaluate and compare it simultaneously. For example, if a skier wants to compare his performance with the previous ones, this function provides visual comparison methods effectively and he can consider the difference among performances. The final step results the scoring. This has three screens illustrated in Fig. 6(c)-(e); tempo, dynamic/symmetry and score, respectively. The tempo screen shows the differences among the target and the actual tempos acquired by performances. The example shows two tempo graphs at a time. The dynamic/symmetry screen shows the symmetry diagram. It represents visually the difference of dynamicity among performances. The score screen shows a triangle where the corners represent the scores of tempo, the symmetry (the average of balance ratio and the balance angle) and the dynamicity respectively. When the score becomes high, the triangle shapes large. The shape of the triangle intuitively informs the skier the lack of skills. The example screen shows the messages in Japanese language mode.

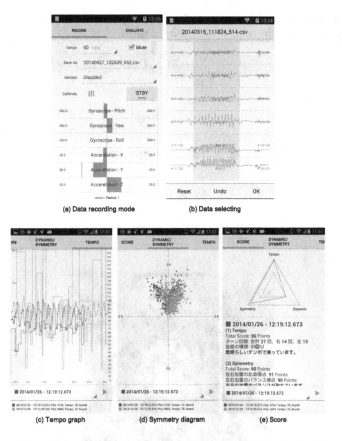

Fig. 6. Screenshots of the ski trainer system implemented on an Android smartphone.

4   Evaluation

We have asked a middle level skier to use the ski trainer who has 10 year experience of skiing, but who does not have tried any qualification tests for any ski licenses. We compare his performance before and after we apply him the ski trainer by comparing twice on two different days. He wear the smartphone in his back as shown in Fig. 7 and he heard the target tempo from a noise canceling earphone. Figures 8(a) and 9(a) show the results from the ski trainer on the first trial day of the skier. After considering the messages and graphs outputted from the ski trainer, his skill level on the second day has become higher such as Figs. 8(b) and 9(b). It becomes better performance when the score and messages from the ski trainer are applied as advice to him. Let us compare the effect of the ski trainer quantitatively among the tempo, the symmetry and the dynamicity.

Table 1. Tempo data $T(i)$ before and after applying the ski trainer. The i in the first column corresponds to the sequence number of turns.

i	$T_{before}(i)$	$T_{after}(i)$
1	35	42
2	140	49
3	20	69
...	...	...
23	140	75
...	...	N/A
33	49	N/A
ρ	47.0	9.8
Score	54	90

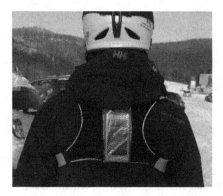

Fig. 7. Wearing the ski trainer piggybacked by a holster small backpack.

– Tempo

As we can see in Fig. 8, the tempo has become stable due to the effort of the skier on the 2nd day. His target tempo is 70. He tried to make the score high following the message from the ski trainer system. Table 1 shows a part of the tempo data calculated from the tempo graph. The score before using the ski trainer was 54. However, he improved his skill to 90. Therefore, we have confirmed that this method provides an effective training to guide the timing related matters of ski's parallel turn. The skier tries to glide any slope by following the target tempo. As the result, the trials raise the skill to turn in any snow environment.

– Symmetry

Before applying the ski trainer system, the skier tends to use the ski edge in the right side mainly because his dominant leg is the right side. Therefore,

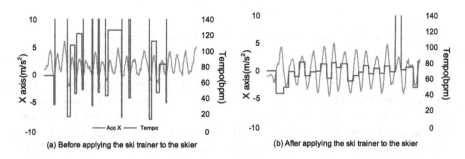

(a) Before applying the ski trainer to the skier   (b) After applying the ski trainer to the skier

Fig. 8. Performance comparison regarding the tempo before and after applying the ski trainer.

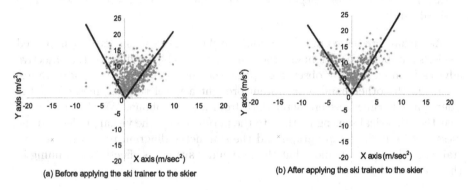

(a) Before applying the ski trainer to the skier   (b) After applying the ski trainer to the skier

Fig. 9. Performance comparison regarding the symmetry/dynamicity before and after applying the ski trainer.

the right side of the vertical axis in the symmetry graph of Fig. 9(a) includes the larger number of points comparing to the left side. The numbers of the points in the right and the left sides of the vertical axis in the graph are 3658 and 1342 respectively. This result causes the balance ratio a bad result. The score was 54. Moreover, the balance angle shows also inclination to the right side. The angles of the approximation lines are also 2.1 and 2.8 in the right and the left sides of the vertical axis respectively. The score was 67. On the other hand, after the participant skier trained himself to correct his performance referring the symmetry diagram of the ski trainer, the balance between the right and the left side has become well. The numbers of the points in the right and the left sides of the vertical axis has become 2597 and 2135 respectively. Additionally, the angles of the approximation lines have become 2.6 and 2.4 for the right and the left sides respectively. Thus, the scores of the balance ratio and the balance angle have become 90 and 92 respectively. According to the observation above, we confirmed that the symmetry diagram provides enough information for considering an inclination to a side, and also it intuitively provides a correct training direction regarding the technique for body balance control.

– Dynamicity

The symmetry diagram before applying the ski trainer shows that the dynamicity becomes between 9.7 m/s^2 in the right side and 8.0 m/s^2 in the left side. Therefore, the skier's parallel turn has an inclination to the right side, also was very compact (not dynamic). The score of the dynamicity was 45. Due to the score, the symmetry diagram and the messages from the ski trainer, he has become aware of using the both sides of ski edges and has moved his balance largely to the right and the left sides. Then the dynamicity has become 9.4 m/s^2 and 9.0 m/s^2 on the right and the left sides respectively. The score has become 46. Thus, because the acceleration to the side edges has become large according to the advices from the ski trainer, his parallel turn has become more elegant than before although the scores do not change significantly.

As we have discussed in this section, the ski trainer system actually improved a skier's parallel turn. Originally, the training had to be provided by the objective advices from experts by observing appearance of the parallel turn of a trainee skier. On the other hand, our system brought a novel training method by the skier himself using accelerometer data from a smartphone. We also confirmed that the numerical scoring method to the performance, the visual guides and the messages from the tempo graph and the symmetry diagram promotes the self-training. Thus, we conclude that the ski trainer system is effective to training in the ski's parallel turns.

4.1   Applying Ski Trainer to Snowboard

We have applied the Ski Trainer system to snowboard. In the case of snowboard, the axes of sensors against the snow slope differ from the ones of ski because the X and the Y axes in Fig. 1 rotated to 90 degree against snow slope. We have asked the same experiments in the previous section to a participant who is high level snowboarder without any qualification license. His snowboarding style is regular (left foot forward).

First, let us see the symmetry diagram as shown in Fig. 10. The turns in the case of snowboard are performed by moving body balance between the back and

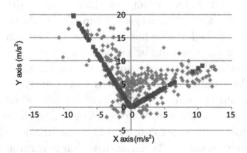

Fig. 10. The symmetry/dynamicity evaluation applying the ski trainer to snowboard.

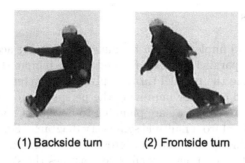

(1) Backside turn   (2) Frontside turn

Fig. 11. The turns of snowboard.

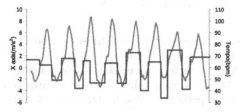

Fig. 12. The tempo evaluation applying the ski trainer to snowboard.

the forth sides. The backside turn Fig. 11(a) uses heel edge of the board. The frontside turn Fig. 11(b) uses toe edge of the board. In the graph, the right side of Y axis plots the accelerometer data during the backside turn. The left side includes the one of the frontside turn. The backside turn has small degree against the snow slope then the frontside turn. Therefore, the graph shows asymmetry and the shape is like an L character. This means that the Ski Trainer system grabs the dynamic posture of the body balance correctly. Using the graph, we are able to observe the objective observation of body balance even when the system is applied in the snowboard.

The tempo graph in the case of snowboard is shown in Fig. 12. The target tempo of the participant was 60 bpm. The upper waves in the graph shows the backside turns. The lower ones are vice versa. The backside turn keeps the tempo in about the target tempo. However, the frontside turn keeps the tempo in about 40 bpm. This means that the tempo during turns between the back and the forth sides become asymmetry in the case of snowboard.

According to the analysis of the graphs mentioned above, the Ski Trainer system acquires the body balance and also the typical physical movement of the snowboard activity. Thus, it is found that possibility to score the skill of the snowboard as the same methods used in the ski's parallel turns. For the future, we are planning to apply the Ski Trainer system to multiple snowboarders among various levels to standardize the skill evaluation.

5   Conclusions

We have designed and implemented a training system using accelerometer on a smartphone for ski's parallel turn. We focused on the tempo, the symmetry and the dynamicity during the parallel turn. Applying the system to a middle level skier, we have a good effect for improving the perspective of his technique. As the next step of this research, we are planning to develop a matching technique to identify the skill level from multiple symmetry diagrams. For example, we will try to match a symmetry diagram to a group of the same diagrams. Then we will design and implement a new system that classifies the skill level to another skier's skill such as an Olympic athlete, and outputs a message such as "Your skill is similar to the gold medalist of this year".

Acknowledgements. This research is partially supported by Tateishi Science and Technology Foundation. And also this work is partially supported by KAKENHI (24240085) Grant-in-Aid for Scientific Research (A). We thank to Prof. Yuji Yamamoto at Nagoya University, Japan for his proofreading of this paper content. We also thank to the participants of the experiments Prof. Kawahara, Prof. Ueno, Dr. Hisamitsu and all other ski experts.

Appendix

The approximation line for the balance angle is calculated using the least squares method. For any accelerometer data of X and Y axis represented by (x_i, y_i) where i is $0 \leq i < N$, we calculate a that makes minimal of;

$$S(a) = \sum (y - ax)^2$$

Because $S'(a) = 0$,

$$\sum xy - a \sum x^2 = 0$$

$$a = \frac{\sum xy}{\sum x^2}$$

The scoring equation for the balance angle uses the data in the right side to calculate a_R and the one of the left side to calculate the a_L. The calculation for the score uses the absolute values of a_R and a_L.

References

1. Federolf, P., Roos, M., Luthi, A., Dual, J.: Finite element simulation of the ski-snow interaction of an alpine ski in a carved turn. Sports Eng. **12**(3), 123–133 (2010)
2. Kondo, A., Doki, H., Hirose, K.: Motion analysis and joint angle measurement of skier gliding on the actual snow field using inertial sensors. Procedia Eng. 6th Asia Pac. Congr. Sports Technol. (APCST) **60**, 307–312 (2013)
3. NONSTOP, August 2014. http://www.nonstopsnow.com/

4. Otsuka, S., Matsuura, K., Gotoda, N., Tanaka, T., Kanenishi, K., Ogata, H., Yano, Y.: Designing the web-community for self-managed training of runners. In: König, A., Dengel, A., Hinkelmann, K., Kise, K., Howlett, R.J., Jain, L.C. (eds.) KES 2011, Part III. LNCS, vol. 6883, pp. 520–528. Springer, Heidelberg (2011)
5. Yoneyama, T., Scott, N., Kagawa, H.: Timing of force application and joint angles during a long ski turn. In: Moritz, E., Haake, S. (eds.), The Engineering of Sport 6, pp. 293–298. Springer, New York (2006)

Monocular Tracking of Human Motion in Evaluation of Hurdle Clearance

Tomasz Krzeszowski[1], Krzysztof Przednowek[2]($\boxtimes$), Janusz Iskra[3],
and Krzysztof Wiktorowicz[1]

[1] Faculty of Electrical and Computer Engineering,
Rzeszów University of Technology, Wincentego Pola 2, 35-959 Rzeszów, Poland
{tkrzeszo,kwiktor}@prz.edu.pl
[2] Faculty of Physical Education, University of Rzeszów,
Towarnickiego 3, 35-959 Rzeszów, Poland
krzprz@ur.edu.pl
[3] Faculty of Physical Education and Physiotherapy,
Opole University of Technology, Prószkowska 76, 45-758 Opole, Poland
j.iskra@awf.katowice.pl

Abstract. In this paper, markerless method of human motion tracking for measurement of hurdle clearance kinematic parameters was presented. The analysis involved 5 hurdlers at various training levels. Acquisition of video sequences was carried out under simulated starting conditions of a 110 m hurdle race. Kinematic parameters were determined based on the analysis of images recorded with a 100 Hz monocular camera. The accuracy of determined hurdle clearance parameters was verified by comparison of estimated poses with the ground truth poses. As the quality criterion, the mean absolute error was adopted. The level of computed errors showed that the presented method can be used for estimation of hurdle clearance kinematic parameters.

Keywords: Hurdle clearance · Markerless human motion tracking · Particle swarm optimization · Monocular camera

1 Introduction

Hurdling is a group of athletic events in which technical preparation plays a significant role. The most prominent hurdles events are 100 meters hurdles (women), 110 meters hurdles (men) and 400 meters hurdles (both sexes). These three distances are all contested at the Summer Olympics and the World Championships in Athletics. The hurdle race technique involves running over 10 hurdles that are from 0.84 to 1.07 m high (depending on the particular event). In those races, the estimation of technique is focused mainly on evaluation of particular hurdles passing stages. Those stages are a complex form of dynamic motion [7]. The existing kinematic studies of hurdle races include mostly the analysis of selected parts of race. The most commonly analysed race element is the so-called "hurdle clearance" [2,3,12]. Among the above-mentioned studies, the most interesting is

© Springer International Publishing Switzerland 2015
J. Cabri et al. (Eds.): icSPORTS 2014, CCIS 556, pp. 16–29, 2015.
DOI: 10.1007/978-3-319-25249-0_2

the research conducted by Čoh [2] describing the technique of running over the hurdle used by the world-record holder Colin Jackson. The kinematic 3D analysis regarded the run over the fourth and fifth hurdle. It was carried out using the ARIEL (Ariel Dynamics Inc., USA) tool. The video material was recorded with two 50 Hz cameras. The conducted research allowed for an accurate determination of the selected kinematic parameters of hurdle clearance. The same author also described a biomechanical analysis of the 100 meters hurdles performed by Brigita Bukovec, the medallist of the Olympic Games in Atlanta [4]. In this paper, kinematic and kinetic analysis of parameters of start, starting acceleration up to the first hurdle, the velocity dynamics between the hurdles and the technique of taking the sixth hurdle were estimated. In study a 2D video system (Ariel Performance Analysis System) was used. The all sequences were recorded with three synchronized cameras with a frequency of 50 Hz. In paper [12] McDonald performed a detailed analysis of the angular momentum of hurdle clearance and presented the assumptions that can help in obtaining minimal loss of forward velocity during hurdle clearance. Another paper describes the study concerning 3D biomechanical analysis of sprint hurdles [16]. To estimate the parameters "Kine analysis" software and two cameras with frame rate of 25 fps were used. The study involved two groups of men and two groups of women at different levels of training. The main objective of the study was to determine the level and comparison of selected kinematic parameters in the analysed groups.

In the biomechanical research of sports events, various computer vision methods play a more and more important role. Motion detection and tracking methods are used among others in analysis of athletic jumps [13,15]. Chinese researchers [21] suggested using computer vision for technique evaluation of athletes jumping on a trampoline. Another solution that uses computer vision techniques is system for tracking players in indoor team games, e.g. handball [14]. The next study [20] presented a motion analysis system of soccer games. The main goal of this paper was to evaluate the teamwork quantitatively based on movement of the players in game. In [19] Sim and Sundaraj proposed the use of optical flow and template matching in markerless human motion analysis. They focused on tracking major body parts of professional golfer directly from a sports broadcast video. Another study proposes motion tracking of a tennis racket using a monocular camera and markerless technique [6]. Whereas the work by [17] makes use of a markerless motion capture system to test for kinematic differences at the lower back, shoulder, elbow, wrist, and racquet between the flat, kick, and slice serves. In the study, seven male NCAA Division 1 players were tested on an outdoor court in daylight conditions. The next application showed that the periodic motion descriptor can successfully classify four sports types: sprint, long-distance running, hurdling and canoeing. The experimental results were performed using video material from the 1992 Barcelona Olympic Games [1].

In this paper, the markerless method of human motion tracking was used; it makes it possible to obtain kinematic parameters for hurdle clearance analysis. These parameters are crucial in the evaluation of hurdlers technique. Correct technique to overcome hurdle is a basic element of motor potential hurdler and does not expose athlete to frequent injuries (frequent in this competition). Properly selected exercises can be also use as a part of physioprevention in this complex athletics competition. The above-mentioned parameters are determined based on the analysis of the sequence of images captured with a monocular camera. An important aspect is the fact, that the suggested method does not involve using any special clothes, markers or other estimation support techniques. To the best of our knowledge, this is the first attempt to measure of hurdle clearance kinematic parameters with markerless motion tracking algorithm.

2   Articulated Human Motion Tracking

The purpose of tracking is to determine the current pose of a human body which reflects as closely as possible to the real pose. It should be noted that capturing the three-dimensional position of a human body is a very difficult task that requires complicated computations [8,11]. The main problems include: high dimensional search space that in issues involving motion tracking can comprise of up to some dozen dimensions; noise occurring in the image and a large variability in appearance of the tracked humans and environment. A significant problem is also the complexity of human motion and the fact that particular parts of the body often are obscured. The situation gets even more complicated when images from only a monocular camera are available. In such case, problems concerning the depth estimation cause additional difficulty. Research teams solve the above-mentioned issues in many different ways. The most common method is making use of simplified human body models [5,8,10], uniform background [5], and also properly selected clothes of the tracked human body in order to facilitate the determination of distinctive features. In the process of tracking, the particle filter algorithm [18] or its modified versions are often used [5]. Those algorithms require, however, a significant number of particles in order to find the correct solution, what directly impacts the time needed for computations. Therefore, in the human body motion tracking process, particle swarm optimization algorithms [8,9,11], are more and more often used, because they enable a more effective exploration of the search space.

2.1   3D Human Body Model

The 3D model is used for simulation of human body motion and determination of its current pose, i.e. position and orientation in space as well as the angles between the joints. The model used in this research is based on the kinematic tree structure consisting of 11 segments; each of them is represented using a truncated cone [5,10], see Fig. 1. The space, in that the model operates, is determined by the number of degrees of freedom (DoF). Each segment can include up to three DoFs that define its orientation; an exception is the pelvis that can contain three additional segments defining the model translation. For tracking the human body motion, models for which the number of DoFs ranges from 26 [10,11] to over 30 [5] are usually used; the model suggested in this paper includes 17 DoFs. Restriction of the search space is possible, since a specific problem is considered, i.e. application of tracking system in order to obtain data for hurdle clearance

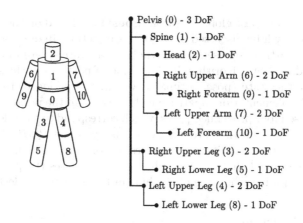

Fig. 1. 3D human body model (left), hierarchical structure (right).

over the distance of 110 m. If you know how the tracked human body would move, you will be able to make some additional assumptions. For example, you can assume that the hurdle runner will move perpendicularly to the camera and will not change its direction. The use of similar assumptions allowed for a significant reduction of the search space, which has a great influence on the complexity of the problem under consideration. The discussed model is fully customizable, and its parametrisation includes a hierarchical structure as well as the length and width of the individual segments. At the moment, both the model configuration and pose of the human body in the first frame of a sequence of images are selected manually.

2.2 Tracking Algorithm

In the motion tracking process, the particle swarm optimization algorithm (PSO) [9], was used; its usefulness in solving problems related to the estimation of human pose has been repeatedly confirmed [8,10,11]. In that algorithm, particle swarm is used in order to find the best solution; each of the particles represents a hypothetical solution of the problem. During the estimation, particles explore the search space and exchange information. In the ordinary PSO algorithm each i-th particle contains the current position $\mathbf{x}_i$, velocity $\mathbf{v}_i$, and its best position $\mathbf{pbest}_i$. Moreover, the particles have access to the best global position $\mathbf{gbest}$, which has been found by any particle in the swarm. The d-th component of velocity and position of each particle are updated based on the following equations:

$$v_{i,d}^{k+1} = \omega[v_{i,d}^k + c_1 r_{1,d}(pbest_{i,d} - x_{i,d}^k) + c_2 r_{2,d}(gbest_d - x_{i,d}^k)], \qquad (1)$$

$$x_{i,d}^{k+1} = x_{i,d}^k + v_{i,d}^{k+1}, \qquad (2)$$

where ω is constriction factor, c_1, c_2 are positive constants and $r_{1,d}$, $r_{2,d}$ are uniformly distributed random numbers. Selection of the best position for i-th particle (**pbest**$_i$) and best global position (**gbest**) are based on the fitness function value, which will be discussed in the next subsection. In our application the position of i-th particle represents the hypothetical state (pose) of an athlete.

In the standard PSO algorithm, initialization of particles in the swarm takes place based on the state (pose) estimated within the period of time $t - 1$. In the suggested implementation, apart from the pose from the period of time $t - 1$ there are also used four predefined poses, which correspond to the selected phases that are characteristic for the hurdle clearance analysis (see P_2, P_3, P_4 and P_5 on Fig. 3). The introduced modification enables a more precise estimation in case of the above-mentioned characteristic phases and increases the probability of a correct pose estimation when one of the human body parts gets lost.

2.3 Fitness Function

The fitness function formulate the degree of similarity between the real and the estimated human pose. The fitness function used in this study is based on two components of the sum. The first of them is determined based on the extracted human silhouette, whereas the other one was based on the edge distance map [8,10]. The value of the function is determined based on the following equation:

$$f(\mathbf{x}) = 1 - (af_1(\mathbf{x}) + bf_2(\mathbf{x})), \tag{3}$$

where $\mathbf{x}$ is the human body pose and a, b are experimentally chosen weighting factors. The $f_1(\mathbf{x})$ function defines the degree of overlap of the rendered 3D model with the extracted silhouette, whereas $f_2(\mathbf{x})$ is determined by comparison of the 3D model edges with the image, including the map with pixel distances from the nearest edge. Figure 2 presents exemplary images with the extracted person.

For human silhouette extraction (Fig. 2(b)) the background subtraction algorithm [22] was used. The second image used in the fitness function, i.e. the edge distance map (Fig. 2(e)), is determined based on the image with extracted edges (Fig. 2(c)), from which edges not belonging to the tracked human body were removed (Fig. 2(d)).

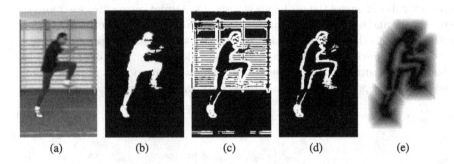

    (a)   (b)   (c)   (d)   (e)

Fig. 2. Person extraction: (a) - input image, (b) - foreground, (c) - edges, (d) - masked edges, (e) - edge distance map.

2.4   Data Collection

The analysis involved five hurdlers at different training levels. Among recorded contestants there was a four times Polish runner-up and twice Polish Youth Champion at 400 meters hurdles. The study was carried out at sports facilities at Opole University of Technology. Registration was made in the athletics hall with four tartan tracks. Throughout the research, the sequence of passing the fourth hurdle in the regulation conditions of 110 m race (height: 1.067 m, distance between the hurdles: 9.14 m) was captured. As shown in the previous studies [2], according to the race speed curve, the speed between the third and fifth hurdle is the greatest and the technique of passing the hurdles is independent of the low start difficulty and increasing fatigue. The analysis included 21 parameters that are presented in Fig. 3. The parameters were selected based on the literature review [2,3,7]. In the analysis, 13 distance parameters and eight angle parameters were taken into account. The description of the specified parameters is shown in Table 1. The sequences were captured with industrial 100 Hz Basler Ace acA645-100gc camera.

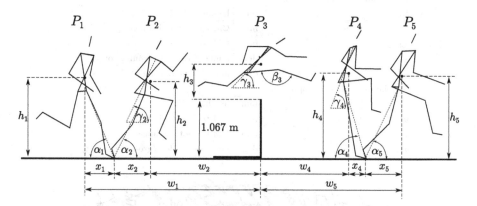

Fig. 3. Hurdle clearance: P_1 - take-off phase (braking), P_2 - take-off phase (propulsion), P_3 - flight phase, P_4 - landing phase (braking), P_5 - landing phase (propulsion).

3   Experimental Results

The markerless motion tracking method was evaluated on five video sequences with hurdle runners. The quality of tracking was made by analyses carried out both through qualitative visual evaluations as well as using of ground truth data. Ground truth data were obtained by manually matching 3D model to athletes on the images containing of five phases characteristic for hurdle clearance analysis (Fig. 3). In Fig. 4 the motion tracking history for the selected athlete was presented. In order to increase the legibility of the generated trace, every fourth recorded frame was presented. The entire sequence was composed of 92 frames,

Table 1. Description of parameters.

Parameter	Unit	Description
P_1 - take-off phase (braking)		
h_1	mm	height of center of mass (CM)
w_1	mm	CM to hurdle distance
x_1	mm	CM to foot distance
α_1	deg	angle of the leg (ground contact)
P_2 - take-off phase (propulsion)		
h_2	mm	height of CM
w_2	mm	CM to hurdle distance
x_2	mm	CM to foot distance
α_2	deg	angle of the leg (ground contact)
γ_2	deg	angle of inclination of the torso
P_3 - flight phase		
h_3	mm	height of CM (over the hurdle)
β_3	deg	angle of the attacking leg
γ_3	deg	angle of inclination of the torso
P_4 - landing phase (braking)		
h_4	mm	height of CM
w_4	mm	CM to hurdle distance
x_4	mm	CM to foot distance
α_4	deg	angle of the leg (ground contact)
γ_4	deg	angle of inclination of the torso
P_5 - landing phase (propulsion)		
h_5	mm	height of CM
w_5	mm	CM to hurdle distance
x_5	mm	CM to foot distance
α_5	deg	angle of the leg (ground contact)

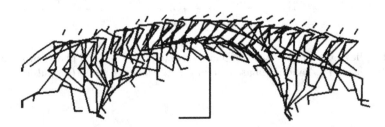

Fig. 4. Motion history for athlete 1, number of frames: 92 (for better readability, only every fourth frame is shown), duration of video sequence: 0.911 s.

which corresponds to the duration 0.911 s. The precise detection of the selected hurdle clearance stages was presented for three chosen athletes (Fig. 5). As one can observe, projected 3D model matches athletes on images reasonably well. From the analysis it follows, that the algorithm provides satisfactory detection of lower limbs whereas there are some problems with estimation of the correct pose of arms. Those problems arise in consequence of the mutual covering of

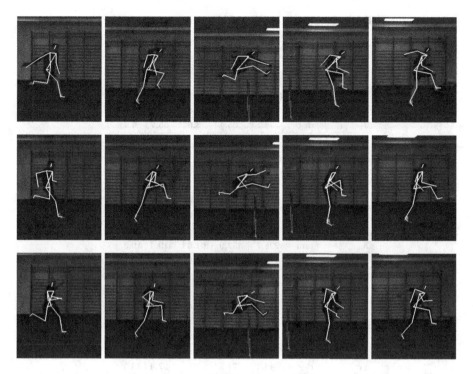

Fig. 5. Tracking results on the three video sequences: first row - athlete 1 in frames #6, 21, 44, 70, 76, second row - athlete 3 in frames #6, 21, 39, 64, 69, third row - athlete 5 in frames #5, 20, 38, 61, 68.

particular parts of body, and they are extremely difficult to eliminate while a monocular camera is used. However, it should be emphasized that in the conducted research, no parameters associated with upper limbs motion were taken into account. In consequence, incorrect arms motion tracking does not impact the measurement of analysed parameters. In the case of lower body there are difficulties in tracking between phases P3 and P4. It may happen that one of the legs is 'lost' (tracking is failed), such a situation can be observed in Fig. 5 for the athlete 5, frame #61. However, due to the use in the process of initializing the particles of four predefined poses (Sect. 2.2), the algorithm is able to correct the error in subsequent frames and estimate the correct posture (Fig. 5, athlete 5, frame #68). Also in this case, the cause of tracking errors are difficulties in estimating the position of a human body pose on the basis of images from a monocular camera.

Numerical characteristics of 21 measured kinematic hurdle clearance parameters are presented in Table 2. This table gives an accurate description of the variables under consideration and their basic statistics, i.e. the arithmetic mean of $\bar{x}$, the minimum value min, the maximum value max, standard deviation sd and coefficient of variation:

$$V = \frac{sd}{\bar{x}} \cdot 100\,\%. \tag{4}$$

Table 2. Characteristics of kinematic parameters.

Parameter	Unit	min	max	sd	$\bar{x}$	V [%]
P_1						
h_1	mm	764.0	1040.0	76.2	927.9	8.2
w_1	mm	2249.0	2741.0	153.8	2551.0	6.0
x_1	mm	239.0	534.5	59.8	378.9	15.8
α_1	deg	46.1	65.4	3.6	55.7	6.4
P_2						
h_2	mm	952.4	1196.0	59.0	1098.0	5.4
w_2	mm	1304.0	1717.0	107.8	1538.0	7.0
x_2	mm	167.3	589.6	104.4	407.3	25.6
α_2	deg	70.2	97.4	7.3	81.1	9.0
γ_2	deg	55.7	81.4	6.3	68.5	9.2
P_3						
h_3	mm	228.7	437.9	61.6	319.4	19.3
β_3	deg	119.9	173.0	14.8	146.6	10.1
γ_3	deg	34.1	56.1	4.7	46.0	10.3
P_4						
h_4	mm	967.2	1193.0	59.4	1093.0	5.4
w_4	mm	1180.0	1486.0	73.1	1344.0	5.4
x_4	mm	18.4	433.2	88.5	236.7	37.4
α_4	deg	15.1	99.4	13.8	81.3	14.0
γ_4	deg	44.1	74.9	7.8	57.4	13.5
P_5						
h_5	mm	903.4	1124.0	63.9	1008.0	6.3
w_5	mm	1663.0	1958.0	73.0	1807.0	4.0
x_5	mm	194.6	811.7	109.7	606.5	18.1
α_5	deg	54.5	94.3	7.7	68.2	11.4

The analysis shows that the average length of hurdle clearance was approximately 3525.2 mm (x_2, w_2, x_4, w_4). The taking off distance was 364.6 mm longer than the landing distance. The trunk inclination angle in landing position was at the level of 57.4°. The greatest variability was observed for distance parameters between the center of gravity and the spot where the foot touched the ground. The measured values are consistent with the sport level of the researched group.

The next step included determination of the error level of particular parameters. Values computed by using the implemented algorithm were compared with the values of the theoretical ground truth reference model (model manually adjusted to the analysed images). The quality criterion was defined for each parameter as:

$$e_j = |\hat{X}_j - X_j|, \tag{5}$$

$$MAE = \frac{1}{N} \sum_{j=1}^{N} e_j, \tag{6}$$

Table 3. Errors of estimated parameters.

Parameter	Unit	$min(e_j)$	$max(e_j)$	$sd(e_j)$	MAE	$NMAE$ [%]
P_1						
h_1	mm	0.5	95.9	29.0	37.0	13.4
w_1	mm	1.8	58.7	14.6	22.0	4.5
x_1	mm	4.2	113.3	28.3	41.3	14.0
α_1	deg	0.1	7.1	1.8	3.1	16.1
P_2						
h_2	mm	6.5	141.2	30.4	66.8	27.4
w_2	mm	2.9	77.3	18.9	32.3	24.9
x_2	mm	1.8	364.9	83.0	105.2	7.8
α_2	deg	0.1	18.9	5.1	5.5	20.2
γ_2	deg	0.2	9.3	2.4	3.5	13.5
P_3						
h_3	mm	0.6	103.0	25.4	27.1	12.9
β_3	deg	0.4	27.2	5.6	7.0	13.2
γ_3	deg	0.0	12.1	3.4	4.5	20.5
P_4						
h_4	mm	0.7	107.5	26.5	41.2	18.2
w_4	mm	0.7	173.6	44.8	55.7	32.7
x_4	mm	1.8	232.1	63.9	135.5	18.2
α_4	deg	0.5	57.5	9.4	7.6	9.0
γ_4	deg	0.1	25.8	6.9	10.0	32.5
P_5						
h_5	mm	1.2	97.6	27.4	38.4	17.5
w_5	mm	3.9	128.9	30.5	59.3	20.1
x_5	mm	6.1	235.9	56.1	99.0	16.0
α_5	deg	0.1	14.9	3.8	4.0	10.1

where e_j - absolute error, N - total number of data, $\hat{X}_j$ - estimated value (determined by the algorithm), X_j - ground truth value, MAE - mean absolute error. The normalized mean absolute error was calculated from formula:

$$NMAE = \frac{MAE}{max - min} \cdot 100\,\%, \tag{7}$$

where max - maximum value of parameter, min - minimum value of parameter.

Table 3 includes the minimum error $min(e_j)$, maximum error $max(e_j)$, standard deviation $sd(e_j)$ and the average error, defined as MAE and $NMAE$. The error analysis revealed that among all distance parameters, estimation of distance between CM and the spot where the foot is touching the ground at the moment of leaving the hurdle (landing) is determined with the greatest error (x_4). That error was $MAE = 135.5$ mm. It is however, worth noting that for that parameter, the least difference from ground truth was only 1.8 mm. The CM height parameters featured relatively small values of MAE (27.1 − 66.8 mm), the CM distance from the hurdle (w_1) at the P_1 phase was determined with the least error. The accuracy of parameters estimation was also defined by the

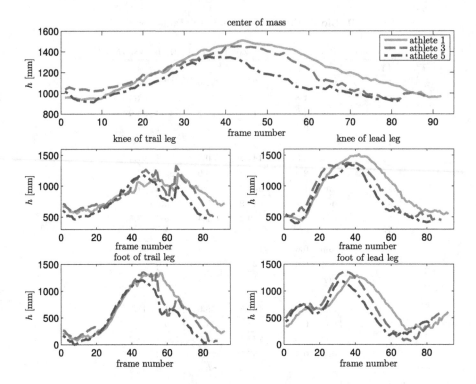

Fig. 6. Trajectory of movement of center of mass, knees and feet for three selected athletes.

MAE error. The angle of the front leg at the 1st stage (α_1) features the least error (3.1°), whereas the trunk angle during landing (γ_4) is determined with the greatest error (10.0°).

The paper focuses on the analysis of five key phases of hurdles clearance, however, the presented algorithm can also be used for the analysis of hurdler's motion during the entire sequence. Figure 6 shows the trajectory of the center of mass, knees and feet for three selected hurdlers. All of the presented trajectories are of similar nature, nevertheless, some differences arising, inter alia, from different body built and technical level of individual athletes can be noticed. For example hurdler 1 shows the highest position of the center of mass for most of the flight and his flight time is the longest (about 50 frames), which can be observed by analysing the trajectory of feet. By contrast the flight time of the fifth athlete is the shortest, approximately 40 frames.

In the analysis of hurdle clearance the velocities of center of mass and swinging leg play an important role [2]. Figure 7 illustrates the velocity of CM during clearing the hurdle by athlete 3, which was characterized by the best hurdle clearance technique. The velocity of center of mass was presented for the five phases (see P_1–P_5 on Fig. 3). The analysis shows that the athlete during take-off phases (P_1 and P_2) accelerates gradually to reach the maximum velocity in the

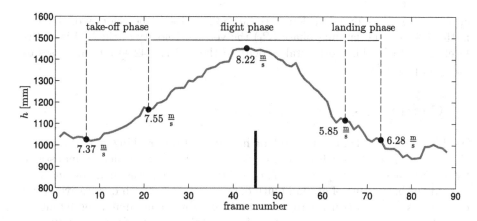

Fig. 7. Velocity of center of mass during clearing the hurdle by athlete 3.

phase of flight. In the next phase it can be observed a decrease in velocity to the value of $5.85 \frac{m}{s}$. In the phase P_5 hurdler accelerates to achieve optimal velocity to overcome next hurdle. Average velocity of CM between phases P_1 and P_5 is equal to $6.93 \frac{m}{s}$.

The velocity components of center of mass and the velocity of swinging leg for take-off and landing phases of athlete 3 was presented on Fig. 8. The horizontal velocity of the CM in the braking phase is $7.35 \frac{m}{s}$ and increases to $7.39 \frac{m}{s}$ in the next phase. In addition to the horizontal velocity of the CM, an important parameter of the P_2 phase is the vertical velocity, which is equal to $1.54 \frac{m}{s}$. The horizontal and vertical velocity determine the elevation velocity of the CM, which is $7.55 \frac{m}{s}$. The velocity of hurdle clearance depends also on the velocity of the swinging leg during the take-off phases [2]. The velocity of the knee of the

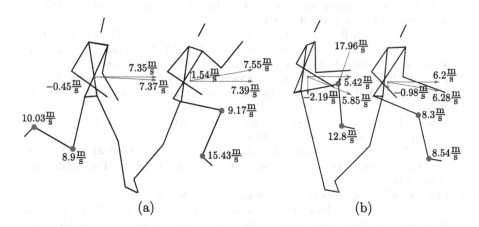

Fig. 8. Velocity components of center of mass and the velocity of swinging leg for athlete 3: (a) - take-off phases (P_1 and P_2), (b) - landing phases (P_4 and P_5).

swinging leg for analysed athlete is equal to 9.17 $\frac{m}{s}$ and the velocity of the foot is 15.43 $\frac{m}{s}$. During landing phase (P_4) the vertical velocity of the CM is at the level of -2.19 $\frac{m}{s}$. The horizontal velocity of the CM is 5.42 $\frac{m}{s}$ and increases to 6.2 $\frac{m}{s}$ in phase P_5.

4   Conclusions

In this paper, markerless method of human motion tracking was presented. Experimental results on five various video sequences of hurdlers demonstrate the effectiveness of the approach. The quality of tracking was made by analyses carried out both using of ground truth data as well as through qualitative visual evaluations. Ground truth data were obtained by manually matching 3D model to athletes on the images. The error analysis justifies the use of presented method for measurement of hurdle clearance kinematic parameters. The proposed system of estimating kinematic parameters can be used in assessing the progress of training and technical preparation of hurdle runners. With a simple method of determining the parameters of hurdle clearance the progress and impact of training means on hurdlers can be monitored. Further work will focus on the use of data obtained for the analysis of more kinematic parameters as well as dynamic parameters of hurdle clearance. In further works a multi-camera system is also going to be tested.

References

1. Cheng, F., Christmas, W., Kittler, J.: Periodic human motion description for sports video databases. In: Proceedings of the Pattern Recognition, 17th International Conference on (ICPR 2004), vol. 3, pp. 870–873. ICPR 2004, IEEE Computer Society, Washington, DC, USA (2004)
2. Čoh, M.: Biomechanical analysis of Colin Jackson's hurdle clearance technique. New Stud. Athletics 1, 33–40 (2003)
3. Čoh, M., Dolenec, A., Tomažin, K., Zvan, M.: Dynamic and kinematic analysis of the hurdle clearance technique. In: Čoh, M. (ed.) Biomechanical Diagnostic Methods in Athletic Training, pp. 109–116. University of Ljubljana (2008)
4. Čoh, M., Kostelic, J., Tomažin, K., Dolenec, A., Pintarič, S.: A biomechanical model of the 100 m hurdles of Brigita Bukovec. Track Coach 142, 4521–4529 (1998)
5. Deutscher, J., Reid, I.: Articulated body motion capture by stochastic search. Int. J. Comput. Vis. 61(2), 185–205 (2005)
6. Elliott, N., Choppin, S., Goodwill, S.R., Allen, T.: Markerless tracking of tennis racket motion using a camera. Procedia Eng. 72, 344–349 (2014). The Engineering of Sport 10
7. Iskra, J.: Scientific research in hurdle races. AWF Katowice (2012)
8. John, V., Trucco, E., Ivekovic, S.: Markerless human articulated tracking using hierarchical particle swarm optimisation. Image Vis. Comput. 28(11), 1530–1547 (2010)

9. Kennedy, J., Eberhart, R.: Particle swarm optimization. In: Proceedings of IEEE International Conference on Neural Networks. vol. 4, pp. 1942–1948. IEEE Press, Piscataway, NJ (1995)

10. Krzeszowski, T., Kwolek, B., Michalczuk, A., Świtoński, A., Josiński, H.: View independent human gait recognition using markerless 3D human motion capture. In: Bolc, L., Tadeusiewicz, R., Chmielewski, L.J., Wojciechowski, K. (eds.) ICCVG 2012. LNCS, vol. 7594, pp. 491–500. Springer, Heidelberg (2012)

11. Kwolek, B., Krzeszowski, T., Gagalowicz, A., Wojciechowski, K., Josinski, H.: Realtime multi-view human motion tracking using particle swarm optimization with resampling. In: Perales, F.J., Fisher, R.B., Moeslund, T.B. (eds.) AMDO 2012. LNCS, vol. 7378, pp. 92–101. Springer, Heidelberg (2012)

12. McDonald, C.: The angular momentum of hurdle clearance. Track Coach **163**, 5191–5204 (2003)

13. Panagiotakis, C., Grinias, I., Tziritas, G.: Automatic human motion analysis and action recognition in athletics videos. In: 14th European Signal Processing Conference Citeseer (2006)

14. Perš, J., Kovacic, S.: A system for tracking players in sports games by computer vision. Elektrotehnični Vestn. **67**(5), 281–288 (2000)

15. Ramasso, E., Panagiotakis, C., Rombaut, M., Pellerin, D., Tziritas, G., et al.: Human shape-motion analysis in athletics videos for coarse to fine action/activity recognition using transferable belief model. Electro. Lett. Comput. Vis. Image Anal. **7**(4), 32–50 (2009)

16. Salo, A., Grimshaw, P.N., Marar, L.: 3-D biomechanical analysis of sprint hurdles at different competitive levels. Med. Sci. Sports Exerc. **29**(2), 231–237 (1997)

17. Sheets, A.L., Abrams, G.D., Corazza, S., Safran, M.R., Andriacchi, T.P.: Kinematics differences between the flat, kick, and slice serves measured using a markerless motion capture method. Annal. Biomed. Eng. **39**(12), 3011–3020 (2011)

18. Sidenbladh, H., Black, M.J., Fleet, D.J.: Stochastic tracking of 3D human figures using 2D image motion. In: European Conference on Computer Vision, pp. 702–718 (2000)

19. Sim, K., Sundaraj, K.: Human motion tracking on broadcast golf swing video using optical flow and template matching. In: 2010 International Conference on Computer Applications and Industrial Electronics (ICCAIE), pp. 169–173, December 2010

20. Taki, T., Hasegawa, J., Fukumura, T.: Development of motion analysis system for quantitative evaluation of teamwork in soccer games. In: Proceedings of the International Conference on Image Processing, vol. 3, pp. 815–818, September 1996

21. Xian-jie, Q., Zhao-qi, W., Shi-hong, X.: A novel computer vision technique used on sport video. In: The 12th International Conference in Central Europe on Computer Graphics. UNION Agency-Science Press (2004)

22. Zivkovic, Z., van der Heijden, F.: Efficient adaptive density estimation per image pixel for the task of background subtraction. Pattern Recogn. Lett. **27**(7), 773–780 (2006)

Prediction of the Results in 400-Metres Hurdles in Two Different Time Intervals Using Statistical Learning Methods

Krzysztof Przednowek[1]($\boxtimes$), Janusz Iskra[2], and Karolina H. Przednowek[1]

[1] Faculty of Physical Education, University of Rzeszów,
Towarnickiego 3, 35-959 Rzeszów, Poland
{krzprz,karprzed}@ur.edu.pl
[2] Faculty of Physical Education and Physiotherapy,
Opole University of Technology, Prószkowska 76, 45-758 Opole, Poland
j.iskra@awf.katowice.pl

Abstract. This research presents the selected statistical learning methods in predicting the results of 400 m hurdles in two different time intervals. The calculated models predict results in selected training period and in annual training cycle. In the study, detailed training programs of 21 Polish hurdlers were analyzed. Building of the predictive models was conducted by means of regression shrinkage and artificial neural networks. To evaluate calculated models the leave-one-out cross validation was used. The outcome of the studies shows that the best method in both analysed time intervals was LASSO regression. The prediction error for a training period was at the level of 0.67 s, whereas for the annual training cycle was at the level of 0.39 s. Additionally, for both time intervals the optimal set of predictors was calculated. In terms of training periods, the LASSO model eliminated 8 variables, whereas in terms of the annual training cycle 12 variables were eliminated.

Keywords: 400 m hurdles · Statistical learning · Predictive models

1 Introduction

Nowadays the sport is an interdisciplinary field. The competitors and coaches have been looking for new solutions to support the training process. One of aspects of training support is using methods of statistical learning. These methods can be used to calculate models which facilitate description of complex training process. They can also help to notice interrelations between the training load and the final result.

Sports prediction involves many forms including predicting sporting talent [13,16] or the prediction of performance results [10,15]. Models predicting sports scores, taking into account the seasonal statistics of each team, are also constructed [6].

The use of regression models in athletics was described by Maszczyk et al. [10], where the model implementing the prediction of results in a javelin throw

© Springer International Publishing Switzerland 2015
J. Cabri et al. (Eds.): icSPORTS 2014, CCIS 556, pp. 30–41, 2015.
DOI: 10.1007/978-3-319-25249-0_3

was presented. The constructed model was used as a tool to support the choice and selection of prospective javelin throwers. On the basis of the selected set of input variables the distance of a javelin throw was predicted. The presented models were classic multiple regression models, and to select input variables Hellwigs method was used.

Another application used in walking races was regressions estimating the levels of the selected physiological parameters and the results over distances of 5, 10, 20 and 50 km [4]. Calculated models were used to develop nomograms. The regressions applied were the classical OLS models, and the coefficient R^2 was chosen for the quality criterion. The study included 45 men and 23 women. The amount of registered data was changed depending on the implemented task and ranged from 21 to 68 models.

Chatterjee et al. [3] have calculated a nonlinear regression equation to predict the maximal aerobic capacity of footballers. The data, on the basis of which the models were calculated, came from 35 young players aged from 14 to 16. The experiment was to verify the use of the test of 20 m MST (Multi Stage Shuttle Run Test) in assessing the performance of VO_{2max}.

Roczniok et al. [16] used a regression equation to identify the talent of young hockey players. The study involved 60 boys aged between 15 and 16, who participated in selection camps. The applied regression model classified individual candidates for future training based on selected parameters of the player. The classification method used was logistic regression. A group of nonlinear predictive models used in sport also supplement the selected methods of 'data mining'. Ofoghi et al. [12] has reviewed the different aspects of the application 'data mining' in sports science.

The significant role is played also by fuzzy expert systems. Practical application of such a system has been described in the work by Papic et al. [13]. The presented system used the knowledge of experts in the field of sport, as well as the data obtained as a result of a number of motor tests. The model based on the candidates data suggested the most suitable sport. This tool was designed to help to search for prospective sports talents.

Previous studies also concern the widespread use of artificial neural networks in sports prediction [6]. Artificial neural networks are used to predict sporting talent, to identify handball players tactics or to analyze the effectiveness of the training of swimmers [14]. Numerous studies show the application of neural networks in various aspects of sports training [11,17,18]. These models support the selection of sports, practice control or the planning of training loads.

The main purpose of the research was verification of selected statistical learning methods in prediction result in 400 m hurdles for two different time intervals. The verification was carried out based on training data of athletes running the 400 m hurdles and featuring a very high-level of sport abilities.

2 Materials and Methods

The analysis included 21 Polish hurdlers aged 22.25 ± 1.96 years participating in competitions from 1989 to 2011. The athletes had a high sport level (the result

Table 1. Description of the variables used to construct the models.

Training period	Annual cycle	Description
y	–	Expected 500 m sprint [s]
–	y	Expected result on 400 m hurdles [s]
x_1	x_1	Age (years)
x_2	x_2	Body mass index
x_3	–	Current 500 m sprint [s]
–	x_3	Current result on 400 m hurdles [s]
x_4	–	Period GPP (general preparation period)
x_5	–	Period SPP (special preparation period)
x_6	x_4	Maximal speed [m]
x_7	x_5	Technical speed [m]
x_8	x_6	Technical and speed exercises [m]
x_9	x_7	Speed endurance [m]
x_{10}	x_8	Specific hurdle endurance [m]
x_{11}	x_9	Pace runs [m]
x_{12}	x_{10}	Aerobic endurance [m]
x_{13}	x_{11}	Strength endurance I [m]
x_{14}	x_{12}	Strength endurance II [amount]
x_{15}	x_{13}	General strength of lower limbs [kg]
x_{16}	x_{14}	Directed strength of lower limbs [kg]
x_{17}	x_{15}	Specific strength of lower limbs [kg]
x_{18}	x_{16}	Trunk strength [amount]
x_{19}	x_{17}	Upper body strength [kg]
x_{20}	x_{18}	Explosive strength of lower limbs [amount]
x_{21}	x_{19}	Explosive strength of upper limbs [amount]
x_{22}	x_{20}	Technical exercises – walking pace [min]
x_{23}	x_{21}	Technical exercises – running pace [min]
x_{24}	x_{22}	Runs over 1–3 hurdles [amount]
x_{25}	x_{23}	Runs over 4–7 hurdles [amount]
x_{26}	x_{24}	Runs over 8–12 hurdles [amount]
x_{27}	x_{25}	Hurdle runs in varied rhythm [amount]

over 400 m hurdles: 51.26 ± 1.24 s). They were the part of the Polish National Athletic Team Association representing Poland at the Olympic Games, World and European Championships in junior, youth and senior age categories. The best result over 400 m hurdles in the examined group amounted to 48.19 s. The collected material allowed for the analysis of 144 training plans used in one of the three periods during the annual cycle of training, lasting three months each. The annual training cycle is divided into three equal periods: general preparation, special preparation and the starting period. In the analysis of training periods, 28 variables were used, including 27 independent variables and 1 dependent variable (Table 1).

Another examined time interval was the annual training cycle, in which the training loads were considered as sums of the given training means used throughout the whole macro-cycle. In the annual training cycle, 25 variables were specified. In order to develop models for the annual training cycle, a total of 48 training plans were used.

2.1 Regression Shrinkage Methods

We are considering the problem of constructing a multivariable (multiple) regression model for the set of multiple inputs X_j, $j = 1, ..., p$, and the one output Y. The input variables X_j are called predictors, whereas the output variable Y – a response. We have assumed that it is a linear regression model in the parameters. In OLS regression a popular method of least squares is used [2,7], in which weights are calculated by minimizing the sum of the squared errors. The criterion of performance $J(\mathbf{w})$ takes the form:

$$J(\mathbf{w}) = \sum_{i=1}^{n} (y_i - \sum_{j=1}^{p} x_{ij} w_j)^2, \tag{1}$$

where w_j are unknown weights (parameters) of the model. In ridge regression by Hoerl and Kennard [8] the criterion of performance includes a penalty for increased weights and takes the form:

$$J(\mathbf{w}, \lambda) = \sum_{i=1}^{n} (y_i - \sum_{j=1}^{p} x_{ij} w_j)^2 + \lambda \sum_{j=1}^{p} w_j^2. \tag{2}$$

Parameter $\lambda \geq 0$ decides the size of the penalty: the greater the value λ the bigger the penalty; for $\lambda = 0$ ridge regression is reduced to OLS regression. LASSO regression by Tibshirani [19], similarly to ridge regression, adds to the criterion of performance penalty, where instead of L_2 the norm L_1 is used i.e. the sum of absolute values:

$$J(\mathbf{w}, \lambda) = \sum_{i=1}^{n} (y_i - \sum_{j=1}^{p} x_{ij} w_j)^2 + \lambda \sum_{j=1}^{p} |w_j|. \tag{3}$$

To solve this regression an implementation of the popular LARS algorithm was used (least angle regression) [5]. In the applied algorithm the penalty is decided by s parameter in the range of 0 to 1. The parameter is the fraction of the penalty used in the LASSO. This regression is also used for the selection of input variables. Regression shrinkage models were implemented in GNU R software programming language with additional packages.

2.2 Artificial Neural Networks

In order to build the predictive model, artificial neural networks (ANN) were also used. Two types of ANNs were applied: a multi-layer perceptron (MLP) and networks with radial basis functions (RBF) [2].

The multi-layer perceptron is the most common type of neural network. In 3-layer multiple-input-one-output network the calculation of the output is performed in feed-forward architecture. Network teaching was implemented by the BFGS (Broyden- Fletcher-Goldfarb-Shanno) algorithm, which is a strong second-order algorithm. During MLP training exponential and hyperbolic tangent function were used as the activation functions of hidden neurons. All the analysed networks have only one hidden layer.

The problem with MLP network is that it can be overtrained which means good fitting to data, but poor predictive (generalization) ability. To avoid this the number m of hidden neurons, which is a free parameter, should be determined to give the best predictive performance. In the RBF network we use the concept of radial basis function. The model of linear regression is extended by considering linear combinations of nonlinear functions of the predictors in the form:

$$\hat{y}_i = \sum_{j=1}^{p} \phi_j(x_{ij})w_j, \tag{4}$$

where $\phi = [\phi_1, \ldots, \phi_p]^T$ is a vector of so called basis functions. If we use nonlinear basis functions, we get the nonlinear model which is, however, a linear function of parameters. The feature of RBF network is the fact that the hidden neuron performs a radial basis function. To implement MLP and RBF the Statistica 10 program was used along with the Automatic Statistica Neural Network.

2.3   Evaluation of Models

In order to select the best model the method of cross-validation (CV) [1] was applied. In this method, the data set is divided into two subsets: learning and testing (validation). The first of them is used to build the model, and the second to evaluate its quality. In this article, due to the small amount of data, leave-one-out cross-validation, (LOOCV) was chosen, in which a test set is composed of a selected pair of data (x_i, y_i), and the number of tests is equal to the number of data n. As an indicator of the quality of the model the root of the mean square error ($RMSE_{CV}$) was calculated from formula:

$$RMSE_{CV} = \sqrt{\frac{1}{n}\sum_{i=1}^{n}(y_i - \hat{y}_{-i})^2}, \tag{5}$$

where: $\hat{y}_{-i}$ – the output value of the model built in the i-th step of cross-validation based on a data set containing no testing pair (x_i, y_i).

3   Result and Discussion

3.1   Prediction in Training Periods

Result prediction concerning the training period for 400 m hurdles involves a defined training status indicator, since it is technically impossible to use the running test in 400 m hurdles within each of the analysed annual cycle periods. Therefore, as the training status indicator, the result of a race over a flat distance of 500 m in the particular periods was assumed. The correlation between the result of 500 m and 400 m hurdles within the competition period is very strong ($r_{xy} = 0.84$); apart from that, it demonstrates statistical significance at the level of $\alpha = 0.001$, confirming the validity of assumption of the 500 m race result as a dependent variable in the course of prediction models development.

The development of a predictive model makes it possible to check how the suggested training affects the final result. The basic model is OLS regression, for which the cross-validation error was at the level of $RMSE_{CV} = 0.72$ s. In ridge regression, the λ parameter is chosen; it determines the additional penalty associated with the regression coefficients. In the study, the dependency between the prediction error and the parameter λ changing from 0 to 20 in steps of 0.1 (Fig. 1a) was determined. The smallest error is generated for the model in which the parameter $\lambda = 3$. The cross-validation error for the optimal ridge regression is 0.71 s. It was also noted that at the initial stage of model optimization, along with the increase of penalty parameter, the prediction error slightly decreases, and after reaching the minimum, it increases up to the level of approx. 0.8 s.

In the LASSO model, the s parameter is chosen; its value ranges from 0 to 1 and it determines the imposed penalty. A graph showing the relationship between the s parameter values and the prediction error $RMSE_{CV}$ was drafted (Fig. 1b). The error generated by the optimal LASSO model ($s = 0.76$) was at the level of 0.67 s. From the determined coefficients (Table 2) it follows, that the variables x_2, x_5, x_8, x_{11}, x_{15}, x_{16}, x_{23}, x_{25} are not taken into account in the prediction task in terms of training periods (coefficients equal to 0).

The eliminated training means belong to the group of 'targeted' ones. The results confirm the views prevailing among sport researchers, that in high-qualified training those exercises should be restricted, and the coach should concentrate on special training [9].

Calculation of the best neural model performing the task of result prediction in terms of training period amounts to determination of the number of neurons in the hidden layer and to selection of the optimal function of hidden layer neurons activation. Therefore, the dependency between prediction error and the number of neurons in the hidden layer for each of the analysed networks was determined (Figs. 1c and d).

The first type of network was a multilayer perceptron with the function of hyperbolic tangent activation. Neural networks consisting of from 1 to 20 neurons in the hidden layer were subjected to examination. It can be noted that the smallest prediction error is obtained for 1 neuron in the hidden layer (Fig. 1c). Prediction error for the optimal model is 0.73 s, and it does not improve the result obtained by the LASSO regression model.

Another network is the MLP network with exponential function. The optimal model for exponential activation function includes also 1 neuron in the hidden layer. The prediction error ($RMSE_{CV} = 0.72$ s) is smaller in comparison to hyperbolic tangent function, but it is greater than the LASSO regression model.

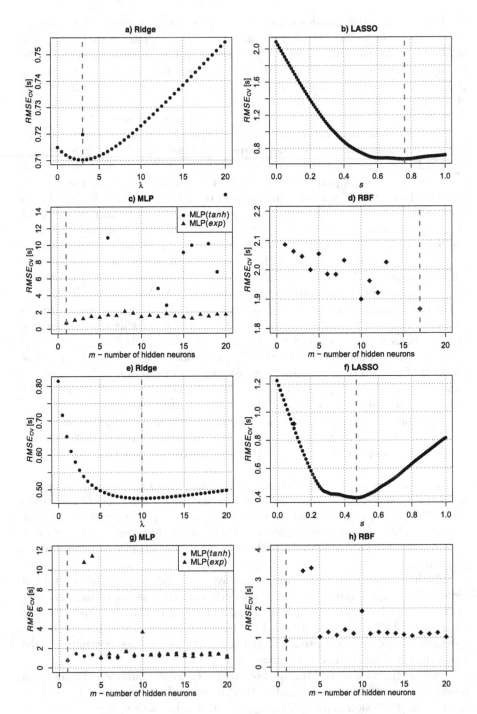

Fig. 1. Prediction error for: (a–d) training period, (e–h) annual training cycle.

Table 2. Coefficients of linear models and error results-training periods.

Regression	OLS	Ridge	LASSO
Intercept	17.5	22.0	15.25
x_1	$-6.43 \cdot 10^{-2}$	$-8.12 \cdot 10^{-2}$	$-5.80 \cdot 10^{-2}$
x_2	$-1.83 \cdot 10^{-2}$	$-4.35 \cdot 10^{-2}$	0
x_3	$7.50 \cdot 10^{-1}$	$6.96 \cdot 10^{-1}$	$7.76 \cdot 10^{-1}$
x_4	$4.85 \cdot 10^{-1}$	$5.11 \cdot 10^{-1}$	$5.62 \cdot 10^{-1}$
x_5	$-9.79 \cdot 10^{-2}$	$-4.03 \cdot 10^{-2}$	0
x_6	$1.28 \cdot 10^{-4}$	$1.29 \cdot 10^{-4}$	$1.86 \cdot 10^{-5}$
x_7	$1.44 \cdot 10^{-4}$	$1.44 \cdot 10^{-4}$	$9.10 \cdot 10^{-5}$
x_8	$-7.75 \cdot 10^{-5}$	$-6.21 \cdot 10^{-5}$	0
x_9	$2.43 \cdot 10^{-7}$	$6.38 \cdot 10^{-8}$	$6.21 \cdot 10^{-7}$
x_{10}	$-9.04 \cdot 10^{-5}$	$-8.98 \cdot 10^{-5}$	$-8.33 \cdot 10^{-5}$
x_{11}	$-2.67 \cdot 10^{-6}$	$-2.39 \cdot 10^{-6}$	0
x_{12}	$1.24 \cdot 10^{-6}$	$1.25 \cdot 10^{-6}$	$5.73 \cdot 10^{-7}$
x_{13}	$-1.51 \cdot 10^{-5}$	$-1.52 \cdot 10^{-5}$	$-1.41 \cdot 10^{-5}$
x_{14}	$-4.47 \cdot 10^{-5}$	$-4.49 \cdot 10^{-5}$	$-2.12 \cdot 10^{-5}$
x_{15}	$5.88 \cdot 10^{-7}$	$1.65 \cdot 10^{-7}$	0
x_{16}	$4.77 \cdot 10^{-6}$	$2.93 \cdot 10^{-6}$	0
x_{17}	$1.31 \cdot 10^{-6}$	$2.58 \cdot 10^{-6}$	$1.26 \cdot 10^{-6}$
x_{18}	$4.19 \cdot 10^{-6}$	$3.48 \cdot 10^{-6}$	$2.14 \cdot 10^{-6}$
x_{19}	$-3.00 \cdot 10^{-5}$	$-2.93 \cdot 10^{-5}$	$-1.05 \cdot 10^{-5}$
x_{20}	$-1.42 \cdot 10^{-3}$	$-1.35 \cdot 10^{-3}$	$-1.00 \cdot 10^{-3}$
x_{21}	$-3.28 \cdot 10^{-4}$	$-4.23 \cdot 10^{-4}$	$-4.00 \cdot 10^{-4}$
x_{22}	$1.13 \cdot 10^{-3}$	$1.34 \cdot 10^{-3}$	$6.00 \cdot 10^{-4}$
x_{23}	$3.94 \cdot 10^{-4}$	$4.74 \cdot 10^{-4}$	0
x_{24}	$-3.82 \cdot 10^{-3}$	$-3.78 \cdot 10^{-3}$	$-1.90 \cdot 10^{-3}$
x_{25}	$-6.10 \cdot 10^{-4}$	$-9.13 \cdot 10^{-4}$	0
x_{26}	$-9.59 \cdot 10^{-4}$	$-1.29 \cdot 10^{-3}$	$-7.00 \cdot 10^{-4}$
x_{27}	$5.68 \cdot 10^{-4}$	$6.34 \cdot 10^{-4}$	$3.00 \cdot 10^{-4}$
$RMSE_{CV}$[s]	0.72	0.71	**0.67**

Similar to MLP networks, RBF network was also subjected to cross-validation. The results are presented in the form of graph, where the prediction error values are shown (Fig. 1d). The optimal RBF model executing the considered task includes 17 neurons in the hidden layer and generates the error of $RMSE_{CV} = 1.9$ s. Errors generated by the RBF network are the greatest among the analysed models.

3.2 Prediction in Annual Training Cycle

OLS model is the basic method applied while seeking optimal solutions for predicting outcome in the annual cycle. The following regression performs this

Table 3. Coefficients of linear models and error results- annual training cycle.

Regression	OLS	Ridge	LASSO
Intercept	31.84	40.30	14.47
x_1	$4.86 \cdot 10^{-1}$	$3.37 \cdot 10^{-1}$	$7.16 \cdot 10^{-1}$
x_2	$-1.08 \cdot 10^{-1}$	$-1.14 \cdot 10^{-1}$	$-9.70 \cdot 10^{-3}$
x_3	$-1.29 \cdot 10^{-1}$	$-1.43 \cdot 10^{-1}$	0
x_4	$4.17 \cdot 10^{-5}$	$4.63 \cdot 10^{-5}$	0
x_5	$7.01 \cdot 10^{-5}$	$1.62 \cdot 10^{-5}$	0
x_6	$-3.58 \cdot 10^{-6}$	$1.36 \cdot 10^{-5}$	0
x_7	$1.86 \cdot 10^{-6}$	$2.36 \cdot 10^{-7}$	$6.12 \cdot 10^{-7}$
x_8	$-1.36 \cdot 10^{-5}$	$-4.63 \cdot 10^{-6}$	0
x_9	$-6.45 \cdot 10^{-7}$	$-3.39 \cdot 10^{-7}$	$3.91 \cdot 10^{-7}$
x_{10}	$-1.31 \cdot 10^{-6}$	$-7.27 \cdot 10^{-7}$	$-5.62 \cdot 10^{-7}$
x_{11}	$1.42 \cdot 10^{-5}$	$1.18 \cdot 10^{-6}$	0
x_{12}	$-1.49 \cdot 10^{-5}$	$-1.87 \cdot 10^{-5}$	$-2.38 \cdot 10^{-6}$
x_{13}	$-2.21 \cdot 10^{-6}$	$-2.34 \cdot 10^{-6}$	$-7.57 \cdot 10^{-7}$
x_{14}	$-6.31 \cdot 10^{-6}$	$-6.23 \cdot 10^{-6}$	$-3.79 \cdot 10^{-6}$
x_{15}	$-1.77 \cdot 10^{-6}$	$-4.41 \cdot 10^{-7}$	0
x_{16}	$-2.82 \cdot 10^{-6}$	$-2.35 \cdot 10^{-6}$	$-4.56 \cdot 10^{-7}$
x_{17}	$1.22 \cdot 10^{-5}$	$8.26 \cdot 10^{-6}$	0
x_{18}	$-9.10 \cdot 10^{-5}$	$-1.90 \cdot 10^{-4}$	0
x_{19}	$2.01 \cdot 10^{-4}$	$-5.91 \cdot 10^{-5}$	0
x_{20}	$1.08 \cdot 10^{-3}$	$1.00 \cdot 10^{-3}$	$5.16 \cdot 10^{-4}$
x_{21}	$1.85 \cdot 10^{-4}$	$1.56 \cdot 10^{-4}$	0
x_{22}	$1.79 \cdot 10^{-3}$	$-1.51 \cdot 10^{-3}$	0
x_{23}	$3.78 \cdot 10^{-3}$	$2.20 \cdot 10^{-3}$	$2,14 \cdot 10^{-3}$
x_{24}	$-3.56 \cdot 10^{-3}$	$-2.06 \cdot 10^{-3}$	$-1.37 \cdot 10^{-3}$
x_{25}	$-3.82 \cdot 10^{-4}$	$-2.47 \cdot 10^{-4}$	$-8.06 \cdot 10^{-5}$
$RMSE_{CV}$ [s]	0.81	0.47	**0.39**

task with error $RMSE_{CV} = 0.81$ s, all the coefficients are different from zero
(Table 3), which means that all the variables form a final result. The analysed
ridge models are regressions for the parameter λ equal from 1 to 20 (Fig. 1e).
The best model was obtained for the parameter $\lambda = 10$. A prediction error generated by the best ridge regression is $RMSE_{CV} = 0.47$ s. Application of this
method has improved by almost a half the capacity of prediction results compared to OLS regression. Ridge regression coefficients, as in the classical model,
are different from zero (Table 3), so all the input variables are involved in the
formation of the projected result. Calculating the optimal LASSO model came
down to analysing models for parameter s from 0 to 1 with a step of 0.01. The
conducted analysis showed that the optimal model is the regression with a parameter $s = 0.47$ (Fig. 1f). This model generates an error of $RMSE_{CV} = 0.39$ s,
which is the best result obtained by linear models. When using this method the
selection of input variables becomes important. The LASSO model, apart from

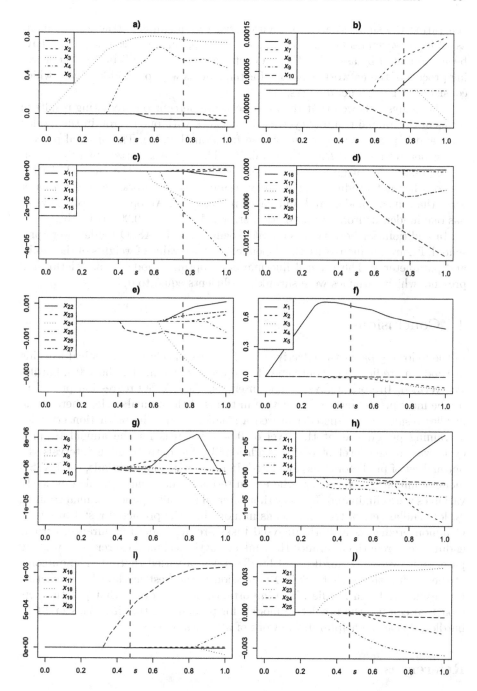

Fig. 2. Coefficients of LASSO regression for: (a–e) training period, (f–j) annual cycle.

generating the smallest error, is characterized by a simpler structure, as many as 12 input variables (x_3, x_4, x_5, x_6, x_8, x_{11}, x_{15}, x_{17}, x_{18}, x_{19}, x_{21}, x_{22}) have been eliminated by assigning them a coefficient equal zero (Table 3). The learning process of the network was done for the models with one hidden layer, which consisted of 1 to 20 neurons respectively.

The analysis showed that the most accurate perceptron predicting results in terms of the annual training cycle is the network with one neuron in the hidden layer and hyperbolic tangent activation function (Fig. 1g). The optimal perceptron generates an error $RMSE_{CV} = 0.74$ s. This result is better than the classical regression, but it gives way to shrinkage models. Using the method of RBF network has not produced satisfactory results. RBF networks generate greater error than linear models and multilayer perceptrons. An optimal RBF network has one hidden neuron and prediction error $RMSE_{CV} = 0.90$ s (Fig. 1h).

In addition, for both time intervals, coefficients of LASSO models were presented. Figure 2 demonstrate the dependence of the value of weights of the model and parameter s. The vertical line marks an optimal model. This relationship presents which variables were shrunk (coefficients equal to 0).

4   Conclusions

In the following paper the effectiveness of the use of selected statistical learning methods in predicting the outcome of competitors training for the 400 m hurdles was verified. In both analysed time intervals, the LASSO regression proved to be the most precise model. Prediction in terms of the annual cycle, where 400 m hurdles result was predicted featured a smaller error. The prediction error for a training period was at the level of 0.67 s, whereas for the annual training cycle was at the level of 0.39 s. Additionally, for both training intervals the optimal set of predictors was calculated. In terms of training periods, the LASSO model eliminated 8 variables, whereas in terms of the annual training cycle, 12 variables were eliminated. In every time interval (training period, annual training cycle), similar sets of training means in modelling the predicted result are used. Common predictors in both analysed tasks are: age, speed endurance, aerobic endurance, strength endurance II, trunk strength, technical exercises — walking pace, runs over 8–12 hurdles and hurdle run in a varied rhythm. The outcome of the studies shows that LASSO regression is the best method for predicting the results in 400 m hurdles. The importance of the work is that practitioners (coaches) can use the predictive models for planning of training loads in 400 m hurdles, its can be helpful in the work of athletics coaches.

References

1. Arlot, S., Celisse, A.: A survey of cross-validation procedures for model selection. Stat. Surv. **4**, 40–79 (2010)
2. Bishop, C.M.: Pattern Recognition and Machine Learning. Springer, New York (2006)

3. Chatterjee, P., Banerjee, A.K., Dasb, P., Debnath, P.: A regression equation to predict VO2max of young football players of Nepal. Int. J. Appl. Sports Sci. **2**, 113–121 (2009)
4. Drake, A., James, R.: Prediction of race walking performance via laboratory and field tests. New Stud. Athletics **23**(4), 35–41 (2009)
5. Efron, B., Hastie, T., Johnstone, I., Tibshirani, R.: Least angle regression (with discussion). Ann. Stat. **32**(2), 407–499 (2004)
6. Haghighat, M., Rastegari, H., Nourafza, N., Branch, N., Esfahan, I.: A review of data mining techniques for result prediction in sports. Adv. Comput. Sci.: An Int. J. **2**(5), 7–12 (2013)
7. Hastie, T., Tibshiranie, R., Friedman, J.: The Elements of Statistical Learning. Springer Series in Statistics, 2nd edn. Springer, New York (2009)
8. Hoerl, A.E., Kennard, R.W.: Ridge regression: biased estimation for nonorthogonal problems. Technometrics **12**(1), 55–67 (1970)
9. Iskra, J., Tataruch, R., Skucha, J.: Advanced training in the hurdles. Opole Univiversity of Technology (2013)
10. Maszczyk, A., Zajac, A., Rygula, I.: A neural Network model approach to athlete selection. Sport Eng. **13**, 83–93 (2011)
11. Maszczyk, A., Roczniok, R., Waskiewicz, Z., Czuba, M., Mikolajec, K., Zajac, A., Stanula, A.: Application of regression and neural models to predict competitive swimming performance. Percept. Mot. Skills **114**(2), 610–626 (2012)
12. Ofoghi, B., Zeleznikow, J., MacMahon, C., Raab, M.: Data mining in elite sports: a review and a framework. Meas. Phys. Edu. Exerc. Sci. **17**(3), 171–186 (2013)
13. Papic, V., Rogulj, N., Plestina, V.: Identification of sport talents using a web-oriented expert system with a fuzzy module. Expert Syst. Appl. **36**(5), 8830–8838 (2009)
14. Pfeiffer, M., Hohmann, A.: Application of neural networks in training science. Hum. Mov. Sci. **31**, 344–359 (2012)
15. Przednowek, K., Wiktorowicz, K.: Prediction of the result in race walking using regularized regression models. J. Theor. Appl. Comput. Sci. **7**(2), 45–58 (2013)
16. Roczniok, R., Maszczyk, A., Stanula, A., Czuba, M., Pietraszewski, P., Kantyka, J., Starzynski, M.: Physiological and physical profiles and on-ice performance approach to predict talent in male youth ice hockey players during draft to hockey team. Isokinetics Exerc. Sci. **21**(2), 121–127 (2013)
17. Rygula, I.: Artificial neural networks as a tool of modeling of training loads. In: Proceedings of the 2005 IEEE Engineering in Medicine and Biology 27th Annual Conference. vol. 1, pp. 2985–2988 (2005)
18. Silva, A.J., Costa, A.M., Oliveira, P.M., Reis, V.M., Saavedra, J., Perl, J., Marinho, D.A.: The use of neural network technology to model swimming performance. J. Sports Sci. Med. **6**(1), 117–125 (2007)
19. Tibshirani, R.: Regression shrinkage and selection via the LASSO. J. Roy. Stat. Soc. **58**(1), 267–288 (1996)

Sampling Rates and Sensor Requirements for Kinematic Assessment During Running Using Foot Mounted IMUs

G.P. Bailey$^{(\boxtimes)}$ and R.K. Harle

Computer Laboratory, University of Cambridge, William Gates Building,
15 JJ Thomson Avenue, Cambridge, Uk
{gpb29,rkh23}@cl.cam.ac.uk

Abstract. Inertial sensors have the potential to enable in-situ monitoring of athletic performance. They may offer applications in injury prevention and rehabilitation as well as in technique assessment for improved performance. This paper investigates the use of foot worn inertial sensors in order to assess running kinematics. Footwear provides a potential platform for continuous and in-situ monitoring that does not require additional components to be worn by the athlete since inertial sensors are now small enough to be integrated into footwear. These sensors are also inexpensive enough to be accessible to consumers, opening up the possibility of biomechanical assessment not only to elite athletes but also recreational runners. To facilitate widespread adoption by athletes of all types, sensor systems must be as cheap as possible. To achieve this, sensor systems must be engineered with sampling rates that are not unnecessarily high and components that are not over specified. At the same time accuracy requirements must be met. We investigate multiple sensor parameters (sampling rate, acceleration range) and the effects these have on the accuracy of kinematic assessment using foot worn inertial sensors. We find that Extended Kalman Filter based trajectory recovery seems to be little affected by sampling rate until lower than 250 Hz. We investigate impact accelerations using an inertial measurement unit attached to the foot and find that, at 250 Hz, the acceleration signal peaks at up to 70g around heel strike. We also show that the addition of a high range accelerometer improves accuracy of two example metrics that may be useful in gait assessment, maximum foot clearance (FC) and mean step velocity (SV). The 95 % limits of agreement for FC using a ($\pm$ 16g) accelerometer were -4.4 cm to 5.4 cm, this was improved using a high range ($\pm$ 200g) accelerometer. The limits of agreement for FC using the improved system where -2.6 cm to 2.6 cm.

Keywords: Running · Gait · Foot kinematics · Continuous sensing · Sampling rates · Sensor requirements · Impact acceleration

1 Introduction

Biomechanical assessment of movement is a complicated but valuable component of today's elite sports training. Assessment of running gait is particularly

© Springer International Publishing Switzerland 2015
J. Cabri et al. (Eds.): icSPORTS 2014, CCIS 556, pp. 42–56, 2015.
DOI: 10.1007/978-3-319-25249-0_4

important and is usually performed within a laboratory setting using video or optical motion capture. These assessments are often characterised by expensive equipment, manual analysis and subjective metrics. Furthermore, the restricted space of a laboratory necessitates evaluation either using a small number of steps or, more often, a treadmill. In neither case is the athlete free to move naturally and there is little guarantee that the gait exhibited is that found in the true sporting arena.

In order to address these issues and to bring kinematic assessment to a wider audience, low-cost inertial sensors are being embedded within consumer products, allowing athletes to be assessed in their natural setting and, additionally, more frequently. In-field constant-assessment brings with it additional benefits, including tracking the progress of injury rehabilitation and enabling longitudinal sports science and biomechanical studies.

Foot-mounted sensors are popular since lightweight sensors can be embedded within shoes in a convenient, unobtrusive way. They may be able to capture rich data, and have already attracted commercial interest (e.g. the Nike+ shoe). In the future, such sensors may be able to track relevant performance metrics or detect compensatory patterns that are the result of poor biomechanics.

Previous studies have shown that foot-worn sensors are capable of providing a full three dimensional trajectory of the foot during steady state running [1] and walking [5] when combined with the inertial strapdown navigation algorithm and methods to reduce the drift associated with inertial navigation techniques. This allows various metrics to be calculated that may be of use to coaches or biomechanists, for example peak foot height or mean step velocity. Our previous work found that usable results could be achieved using both an Extended Kalman Filter and a linear dedrifting technique in combination with the strapdown Algorithm [1]. The work also suggested limitations in the accelerometer resulted in short periods of sensor saturation around heel strike, and that this may have compromised results.

In order to facilitate wider adoption of kinematic sensing, wearable sensor systems used must be as cheap as possible. To achieve this sensor systems should be engineered with sampling rates that are not unnecessarily high and with sensor components that meet the requirements of the task, including required accuracy. Therefore, the purpose of this study is to assess the effect of sensor parameters on the accuracy of tracking the three dimensional trajectory of the foot during steady state running.

We address the following research questions:

- *How do sampling rates affect the accuracy of trajectory recovery?*
  Below a certain point, lower sampling rates might be expected to produce less accurate results. At what point does the sampling rate compromise results? There will be a trade off with sensor requirements.
- *What are the requirements of inertial sensors in terms of range?*
  In order to capture the trajectory of the foot using inertial sensors, the captured signals should not contain periods of saturation. The required range of the sensor will depend on the sampling rate used. For lower sampling rates,

higher frequencies will be attenuated during the low pass filter stage reducing requirements on the sensor. The running surface may also affect the sensor requirements and so we include outdoor running on a variety of surfaces.

– *How much does a small amount of sensor saturation affect results?*
Our previous study found that any sensor saturation usually happens at heel strike and typically only for a few milliseconds [1]. Is it necessary to have a high range inertial sensor or do periods of sensor saturation have minimal affect on the accuracy of the results?

In answering these questions we will structure the paper as follows. A section detailing the experimental platform will be provided, followed by a section for each of the research questions outlined above. These sections will contain methods and results for the experiment required to answer each question. We will conclude by discussing how the results of each of the three experiments trade off.

2   Background

Limited research has been conducted with foot worn sensors for running. However, some studies have looked at impact accelerations at heel strike with sensors attached to the shank. For example, investigation into the effect of fatigue on impact acceleration was undertaken by attaching a $\pm 50g$ accelerometer to the tibial tuberosity [6]. A high sampling rate was used (1667 Hz) and the authors found that the average impact acceleration increased with fatigue to $11.1 \pm 4.2g$. However, impact accelerations at the tibial tuberosity are likely to be much smaller than those present at the foot due to attenuation provided by knee and ankle joints.

Strapdown techniques have previously been investigated for use in assessing running kinematics but sensor saturation was found around heel strike using a $\pm 16g$ sensor at 1 kHz [1]. Another study used a similar technique with a 100 Hz sampling rate but limitations in the video reference system used as ground truth make it difficult to compare the two studies in terms of accuracy [2]. This makes it difficult to assess whether or not a sampling rate of 100 Hz is adequate for kinematic assessment.

For pedestrian localisation applications, optimal sampling frequency has been investigated [7]. Although the authors did investigate a wide range of scenarios including running, they did not evaluate the effects lower sampling rates had on accuracy for running. They concluded from a frequency based analysis that the lowest usable sampling rate for running would be 300 Hz.

3   Sensor Platform and Data Capture

The sensor platform and methods common to each part of the paper will be described in the following section.

3.1   Inertial Sensors

Capture of inertial sensor data was facilitated using the ION (Imperceptible On-body Node) sensor platform [4] with the addition of an Inertial Measurement Unit (IMU) providing a three-axis $\pm 16g$ accelerometer and $\pm 2000°\text{s}^{-1}$ gyroscope (MPU-6000, InvenSense Inc.) and containing an internal 16 bit Analog-Digital Converter (ADC).

Additionally an analogue three-axis accelerometer (ADXL377, Analog Devices Inc.) with a $\pm 200g$ range was included on the same PCB as the MPU-6000, mounted on the reverse side such that both sensors were co-located to expose them to the same motion. The ADXL377 was connected to the ION sensor platform's 14 bit ADC.

The platform was extended to contain two accelerometers due to sensor saturation observed in earlier experiments. The lower $16g$ range sensor was used to capture the majority of the data with the $200g$ sensor capturing the high frequency peaks that occur near heel strike.

The MPU-6000 has an internal Digital Low Pass Filter, meaning the accelerometer and gyroscope signals on the MPU-6000 had a bandwidth of 260 Hz and 256 Hz respectively. The analogue accelerometer was set up with a 500 Hz bandwidth.

All IMU signals were sampled at 1 kHz and logged to on-board flash memory. In all experiments the ION sensor was placed on the lateral side of the shoe in line with the ankle, as seen in Fig. 1. The sensor was firmly taped to the outside of the shoe to simulate the scenario where it was built into the shoe, perhaps embedded in the sole in a similar manner to the Nike+ shoe. The sensor placement is also justified by a study [8] which assessed the validity of the zero-velocity assumption used in foot mounted inertial navigation [3] techniques. The study investigated different mounting locations on the foot and showed that the sensor position we have used is among the best suited to using this assumption [8].

The sensor platform is lightweight, weighing approximately 15 grams in total, including battery.

3.2   Ground Truth

Ground truth, where applicable, was captured using an optical motion capture system (Vicon Motion Systems, UK) sampling at 240 Hz.

For experiments requiring ground truth, a treadmill was used in order to capture many steps in a limited motion capture area. While the biomechanics of treadmill running may be different to overground running, results of this study should also be applicable to kinematic assessment of overground running. This follows from the observation that, from a sensing perspective, treadmill running differs from overground running only in frame of reference.

The treadmill was set up without any inclination as measured with a spirit level. The ION sensor was attached to a custom jig containing 3 retro-reflective markers (Fig. 1) for the motion capture system. The jig adds an additional 30 grams of weight to the system (45 grams total, including ION) but remains

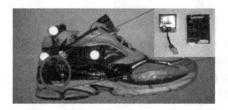

Fig. 1. Shoe with IMU and Jig for facilitating ground truth capture using the Vicon Motion capture system.

comfortable for test runs. The jig was laser cut and the MPU-6000 and retro-reflective markers were aligned with laser-etched outlines to ensure alignment between the jig and the inertial sensor axes.

3.3 Combining Accelerometer Signals

Our previous work shows that for treadmill running at $3.4\,\mathrm{ms}^{-1}$ and below, and at a sampling rate of 1 kHz, sensor saturation is present in the accelerometer signals when a $\pm16g$ accelerometer is in use for short periods of time [1].

Since the majority of the step contains signals within the $16g$ range and only a few samples per step are saturated, the $16g$ accelerometer data was used. Any sensor saturation was corrected for using the $200g$ accelerometer to 'fill-in' the saturated samples. This means that the lower noise and higher resolution (16 bit vs. 14 bit) of the MPU-6000 ($16g$) was utilised for the majority of the step.

The process of combining the accelerometer signals was as follows. In order to avoid any artifacts produced by sensor nonlinearities near the limit of the MPU-6000s range, samples with a value greater than $140\,\mathrm{ms}^{-2}$ were replaced by those from the higher range sensor. When applicable, this replacement was done before any further processing (e.g. down-sampling).

4   Methods and Results

In order to address the research questions outlined in Sect. 1, a number of experiments were designed to test sensor requirements. The methods and results of each experiment are described in this section.

4.1 Effect of Sampling Rates

In order to assess sensor requirements at varying sampling rates, inertial data were collected at a 1 kHz sampling rate before being digitally downsampled to simulate lower sampling rates.

Four participants took part in the study (2 male, 2 female). All participants had a heel-strike running pattern. Ethics committee approval was obtained. Participants were asked to warm up on the treadmill for a few minutes to familiarise themselves with the environment and treadmill speeds. Once the warm up period was complete, the athlete rested for two minutes as the experimental process was explained. Four ninety-second runs were completed, with data logging, by each participant. Data logging included inertial data and motion capture data as described previously. Each run was performed at a predetermined treadmill speed, approximately $2.3\,\mathrm{ms}^{-1}$, $2.7\,\mathrm{ms}^{-1}$, $3.0\,\mathrm{ms}^{-1}$ and $3.4\,\mathrm{ms}^{-1}$, as measured by the Vicon system. Prior to and immediately after each run, the athlete was asked to stamp their feet three times in order to facilitate simple synchronisation between the Vicon and ION systems. A single sensor placed on the right foot was used to conduct the experiment. Due to the acceleration and deceleration of the treadmill at the start and end of each run the middle 90 steps were taken from each run to provide a total of 1440 steps for analysis.

Once data collection was complete the signals were subsequently downsampled in order to simulate lower sampling rates. Integer downsampling factors were used so that interpolation was avoided.

Downsampling for a given downsampling factor, M, proceeded as a two step process. Firstly, to avoid aliasing affects, the data was low-pass filtered. A 4th order butterworth filter was used with a cut off frequency of $0.8 f s_t$ where $f s_t = \frac{f s_b}{M}$ and $f s_t$ is the target sampling rate with $f s_b$ the base sampling rate used by the ION sensor platform (always 1 kHz). Secondly, the resulting signal was decimated by retaining every M^{th} sample.

An Extended Kalman Filter (EKF), paired with an inertial strapdown algorithm, was used to recreate the trajectory of the foot from the inertial data [1,3]. The speed of the treadmill belt was applied as a pseudo measurement during the mid-stance phase of gait along with a zero-foot height pseudo measurement.

As an example of the kind of output that this technique can enable, Fig. 2 contains two example steps from two different people running at the same speed. Differences in technique can be seen between the two in these 2D plots. While 3D plots are possible we use a 2D plot here to make the differences clearer. To provide context for viewing these graphs, Fig. 3 shows 6 frames from high speed video annotated with the trajectory of the foot.

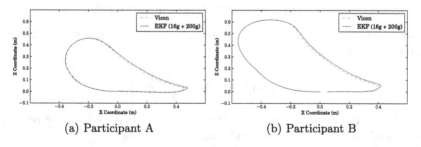

(a) Participant A   (b) Participant B

Fig. 2. 2D plots of position taken from inertial sensor data and ground truth using a motion capture system. The red line represents ground truth and the blue the inertial solution. Both solutions taken from running on a treadmill at $3.4\,\mathrm{ms}^{-1}$ (Color figure online).

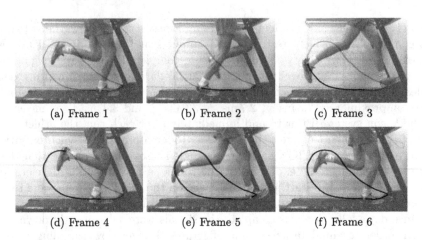

(a) Frame 1   (b) Frame 2   (c) Frame 3

(d) Frame 4   (e) Frame 5   (f) Frame 6

Fig. 3. Six video frames, manually annotated to demonstrate the trajectory of treadmill gait, the right foot is traced in this instance.

This method was applied to each run from each participant at each downsampling factor. The downsampling factors used produced the equivalent of 500 Hz, 250 Hz, 125 Hz, and 62.5 Hz in addition to the 1000 Hz raw signal.

The technique creates a rich set of data detailing the velocity, position and angle of the foot at the time each inertial sample was taken. For trajectory evaluation the position, velocity and attitude error is calculated for each step. Errors are calculated stepwise as offsets in position at the start of the step are irrelevant for an assessment of the step, therefore the ground truth and inertial solutions are aligned in space before calculating the following metrics.

Position error was calculated in the following way:

$$s^{error}(i, k) = \|\mathbf{s}^{inertial}(i, k) - \mathbf{s}^{vicon}(i, k)\| \tag{1}$$

and velocity error was calculated as:

$$v^{error}(i, k) = \|\mathbf{v}^{inertial}(i, k) - \mathbf{v}^{vicon}(i, k)\| \tag{2}$$

where i is the step number and k sample number within step i. Error in attitude was assessed as

$$\theta^{err}(i, k) = \arccos\left(\frac{\mathbf{A}.\mathbf{B}}{\|\mathbf{A}\|\|\mathbf{B}\|}\right) \tag{3}$$

where $\mathbf{A}$ and $\mathbf{B}$ represent the vector $[0, 0, 1]^T$ in the sensor's frame of reference as measured by the INS solution and Vicon respectively.

Figure 4 shows how sampling rates affect the mean error in position, velocity and attitude. The graphs show that with sampling rates lower than 250 Hz the position and velocity error starts to increase rapidly meaning that 1 kHz is unnecessary and in order to reduce sensor requirements a lower sampling rate

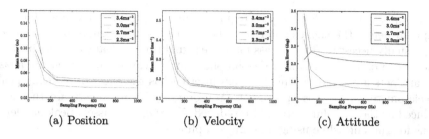

(a) Position   (b) Velocity   (c) Attitude

Fig. 4. Mean error for position, velocity and attitude, for differing sampling rates.

may be used without a large affect on accuracy up to 250 Hz. Attitude errors were not as affected by lower sampling rates staying stable until 125 Hz.

Examples of the full 3D trajectory recovered by the system are shown for two representative steps in Fig. 5 where the lower sampling rate has resulted in much poorer performance.

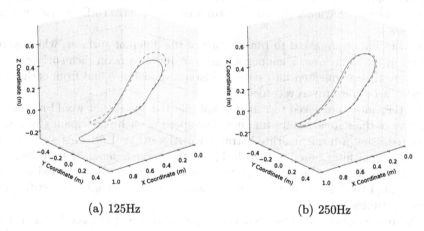

(a) 125Hz   (b) 250Hz

Fig. 5. Figures showing a single step's trajectory recovery at two different sampling rates.

4.2   Sensor Requirements

In order to find optimal sensor parameters we conducted an experiment to determine the requirements for the range of the accelerometer and gyroscope. This is important to make sure that sensors do not saturate during running as this may impair the accuracy of the measurement obtained using strapdown techniques.

Parameters that affect these requirements are sampling rate, running speed and the characteristics of the running surface.

Sampling rates affect sensor requirements due to the low pass filtering required before the signals enter the ADC. Before sensor signals are quantised, it is usually necessary to low-pass filter the signal (in the analogue domain) to a bandwidth of less than half of the sampling rate (Nyquist rate) to ensure aliasing artifacts are avoided. This low-pass filtering has the effect of reducing peak accelerometer and gyroscope signals. Sensor range requirements are therefore reduced as the sampling rate is also reduced. We therefore assess peak accelerations for running while using differing sampling rates.

The accuracy of the algorithms used in [1] to assess running kinematics have, so far, been assessed using a treadmill. While in use, treadmills may flex visibly as the runner hits the treadmill belt. This may reduce the peak accelerations observed at impact. Since the primary use case of such sensing is in overground running outside, we investigated the effect of a number of outdoor surfaces on the sensor range requirements as these are likely to be larger than for a treadmill. For example, impact accelerations on tarmac are likely to be distinct from those of grass or treadmill running.

Accelerometer and gyroscope data were collected for 3 participants (2 male, 1 female) and 5 surfaces. The 5 surfaces tested were picked as likely scenarios for outdoor running. Surfaces chosen were running track, astro turf, tarmac, gravel, and grass.

Participants were asked to run on each of the different surfaces, which were located in the same area. Each participant ran 100 meters on each surface. The data were then segmented into steps, midstance-midstance and from each step the peak acceleration was recorded.

Participants were asked to run at a self-selected speed that would be representative of their steady state running. The speed of each participant's run was estimated using a linear dedrifted strapdown Algorithm [1,5]. This was chosen over a Kalman filter based approach due to the lower number of steps logged. The linear dedrift method does not need time for a filter to settle and so was better suited to these shorter runs with similar levels of accuracy as verified by previous studies.

The results obtained show that the largest factor in peak acceleration was the foot speed but that surface also affected requirements. Figure 6 shows the impact acceleration for all steps logged plotted against the mean foot velocity (SV) for each step. SV was defined as in [5], that is mean velocity in the ground plane (the XY plane). For each step, between midstance events, the following was calculated:

$$SV(i) = \frac{\sum_{k=0}^{N_i} \sqrt{v_x(i,k)^2 + v_y(i,k)^2}}{N_i} \qquad (4)$$

where i is the step number, k is the sample number within step i, and N_i is the number of samples within step i.

Figure 6 shows that even at 62.5 Hz there were a few samples that would saturate a $16g$ sensor at higher speeds. At 1 kHz the majority of steps would

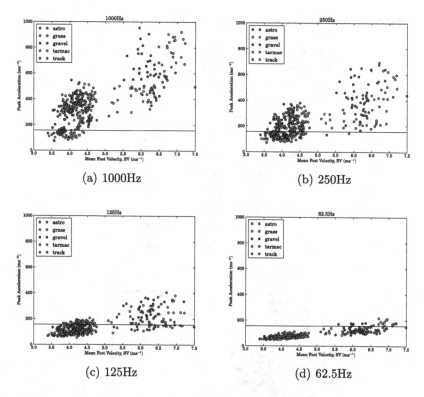

Fig. 6. Figures showing peak acceleration plotted against mean foot speed for each step. The horizontal lines marks the limit of the 16g sensor above which the sensor with a ±16g range would saturate.

show sensor saturation with a 16g sensor and the situation improves only slightly at 250 Hz, the point at which we found the optimal sampling rate.

Mean and maximum peak accelerations are shown in Table 1 showing high maximum accelerations on tarmac of around 90g. Study of peak gyroscope signals were inconclusive as at higher speeds the sensor saturated and it was not possible to obtain a higher range sensor than the ±2000°s^{-1} sensor contained in the MPU-6000. Figure 7 shows the data obtained at the 1 kHz sampling rate, sensor saturation can be seen at higher speeds.

4.3 Effect of Saturation on Measurement Accuracy

While sensor saturation has been suggested as a potential factor that may decrease the accuracy of measurement results no work has yet investigated how significant the loss in accuracy might be. Here we compare the accuracy of results using the 16g accelerometer only, to that which replaces saturated samples with those taken from the 200g accelerometer.

Table 1. Mean and maximum step accelerations for the accelerometer.

Sampling Rate (Hz)	Surface	Mean (ms^{-2})	Max. (ms^{-2})
1000	astro	244	575
	grass	229	503
	gravel	438	954
	tarmac	481	922
	track	430	729
250	astro	207	539
	grass	168	428
	gravel	261	651
	tarmac	286	694
	track	272	635

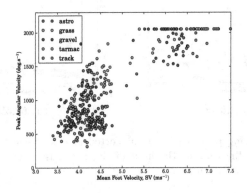

Fig. 7. Plot of maximum rate against mean foot speed showing saturation of the $\pm 2000°\mathrm{s}^{-1}$ gyroscope.

This investigation re-uses the data listed in Sect. 4.1 and the Extended Kalman Filter was applied in the same manner. However the filter was run twice, once with the data as described in Sect. 3.3 and once with data from only the $16g$ accelerometer containing sensor saturation. The data were processed for the highest sampling rate available, 1 kHz.

Error statistics were calculated as in Sect. 4.1 to give error values for each sample in each step. Subsequently, for each step, the maximum and mean errors were calculated for position, velocity and attitude. For example $s_{max}^{error}(i) = max_k(s^{error}(i,k))$ and $s_{mean}^{error}(i) = mean_k(s^{error}(i,k))$ give the maximum error in position and the mean error in position for step i. These statistics were similarly calculated for velocity and attitude. The mean and standard deviation for these statistics are presented in Table 2.

The results show an increase in the error for the $16g$ only trajectory recovery. Table 2 shows the results for the fastest treadmill speed recorded, $3.4\,\mathrm{ms}^{-1}$. It can

Table 2. Mean and standard deviation of per-step metrics for different sensor setups at 1 kHz while running at 3.4 ms^{-1}.

Measurement	Sensor	Mean and SD
s_{max}^{error} (m)	Combined	0.087 ± 0.061
	16g	0.142 ± 0.115
s_{mean}^{error} (m)	Combined	0.048 ± 0.033
	16g	0.079 ± 0.063
v_{max}^{error} (ms^{-1})	Combined	0.52 ± 0.12
	16g	0.60 ± 0.21
v_{mean}^{error} (ms^{-1})	Combined	0.16 ± 0.08
	16g	0.24 ± 0.15
θ_{max}^{error} (Deg)	Combined	3.30 ± 0.90
	16g	4.71 ± 1.85
θ_{mean}^{error} (Deg)	Combined	1.77 ± 0.71
	16g	2.98 ± 1.48

be seen that there is a reduction in the mean and maximal error when using the combined 16g/200g sensor as opposed to 16g only.

As an example of a potentially interesting metric that could be calculated, the mean foot velocity was also assessed over all steps. Mean foot velocity (SV) was calculated as defined in Sect. 4.2.

Bias, standard deviation and 95 % limits of agreement (bias ± 1.96σ) were calculated for the SV metric over all steps for both sensor setups. Using the combined setup the bias and standard deviation were 0.007 ± 0.0156 ms^{-1} with limits of agreement −0.023 ms^{-1} to 0.038 ms^{-1}. Using the 16g only sensor the bias and standard deviation were 0.006 ± 0.020 ms^{-1} with limits of agreement -0.033 ms^{-1} to 0.044 ms^{-1}. Bland-Altman plots for the results can be seen in Fig. 8. Both show some correlation in error with speed and the combined sensor setup shows slightly tighter limits of agreement. However, both sensor setups produce a level of accuracy that may be useful for this metric.

Foot Clearance (FC) [5] was also calculated for both the 16g and Combined sensors for each step. It was calculated as in Eq. 5 and the results are shown in the Bland-Altman plots in Fig. 9.

$$FC(i) = max_k(v_z(i,k)) \qquad (5)$$

The FC results show larger improvements using the combined sensors in comparison to the SV results. The limits of agreement for the 16g only sensor were -4.4 cm to 5.4 cm, this improved using the combined sensors to -2.6 cm to 2.6 cm. Bias for the 16g and combined sensors were 0.5 cm and 0.0 cm respectively, with little evidence of a change in bias with increasing speed in either case.

Examples of error progression over a single step (in both attitude and velocity) can be seen in Figs. 10 and 11. These were taken from one of the participants

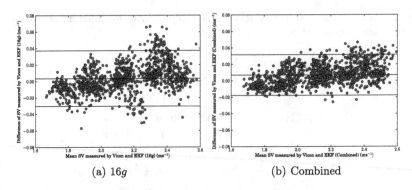

(a) 16g   (b) Combined

Fig. 8. Bland-Altman plots for SV as calculated from Combined and 16g sensor data.

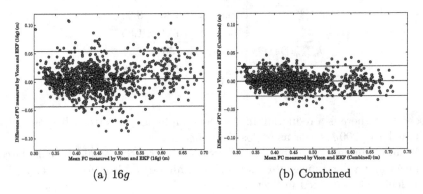

(a) 16g   (b) Combined

Fig. 9. Bland-Altman plots for FC as calculated from Combined and 16g sensor data.

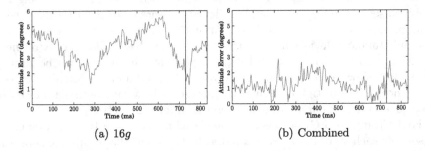

(a) 16g   (b) Combined

Fig. 10. Attitude errors for a representative step from Combined and 16g sensor data. The vertical bar represents the time of heel-strike.

showing a large amount of sensor saturation. The figures show a marked reduction in error. This may suggest that greater benefits will be achieved using combined sensors in faster running while outdoors where higher impact accelerations are expected.

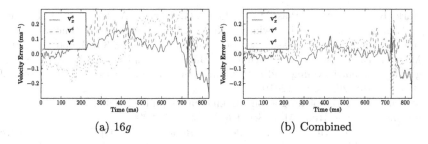

(a) 16*g*   (b) Combined

Fig. 11. Velocity errors for a representative step from Combined and 16*g* sensor data. The vertical bar represents the time of heel-strike.

5   Conclusions

This work has shown that a trade off in sampling rate is possible in order to obtain lower sensor requirements. Extended Kalman Filter based trajectory recovery seems to be little affected by sampling rates until below 250 Hz. However at 250 Hz there would still be regular saturation in overground running on outdoor surfaces using a ±16*g* accelerometer.

We also show that sensor saturation does affect the accuracy of the trajectory recovery. We found that the addition of a high range accelerometer resulted in up to a 40 % reduction in error for some metrics, for example the reduction of mean attitude error reduced from 2.89° to 1.77°. However, it remains unclear how much larger peak accelerations present in higher speeds in an outdoor scenario would affect the accuracy as we were limited in the maximum speed of the treadmill. As such, it remains unclear as to how the method would perform for elite endurance athletes at greater running speeds. Further research should seek to attempt to evaluate these methods at higher speed.

We have been unable to assess requirements for the range in angular velocity measurement to inform gyroscope selection due to limitations in our sensor at higher speeds and it may prove difficult to test in the future due to the lack of commercial availability of MEMS gyroscopes that have a higher range than the one used in this paper ($\pm 2000°\text{s}^{-1}$). Further work may therefore seek to assess whether or not gyroscope saturation has a significant affect on measurement accuracy. If it is found to affect results further work should seek to mitigate these periods of saturation if possible.

References

1. Bailey, G.P., Harle, R.: Assessment of foot kinematics during steady state running using a foot-mounted IMU. Procedia Eng. **72**, 32–37 (2014)
2. Bichler, S., Ogris, G., Kremser, V., Schwab, F., Knott, S., Baca, A.: Towards high-precision IMU/GPS-based stride-parameter determination in an outdoor runners' scenario. Procedia Eng. **34**, 592–597 (2012)
3. Foxlin, E.: Pedestrian tracking with shoe-mounted inertial sensors. IEEE Comput. Graph. Appl. **25**(6), 38–46 (2005)

4. Harle, R., Taherian, S., Pias, M., Coulouris, G., Hopper, A., Cameron, J., Lasenby, J., Kuntze, G., Bezodis, I., Irwin, G., Kerwin, D.G.: Towards real-time profiling of sprints using wearable pressure sensors. Comput. Commun. **35**(6), 650–660 (2011)
5. Mariani, B., Hoskovec, C., Rochat, S., Büla, C., Penders, J., Aminian, K.: 3D gait assessment in young and elderly subjects using foot-worn inertial sensors. J. Biomech. **43**, 2999–3006 (2010)
6. Mizrahi, J.: Effect of fatigue on leg kinematics and impact acceleration in long distance running. Hum. Mov. Sci. **19**(2), 139–151 (2000)
7. Munoz Diaz, E., Heirich, O., Khider, M., Robertson, P.: Optimal sampling frequency and bias error modeling for foot-mounted IMUs. In: International Conference on Indoor Positioning and Indoor Navigation, pp. 1–9. IEEE, October 2013
8. Peruzzi, A., Della Croce, U., Cereatti, A.: Estimation of stride length in level walking using an inertial measurement unit attached to the foot: a validation of the zero velocity assumption during stance. J. Biomech. **44**, 1991–1994 (2011)

A Real-Time Simulator of Foiling Catamarans

Paolo Conti$^{(\boxtimes)}$ and Filippo Rocchini

Department of Engineering, University of Perugia, Perugia, Italy
`paolo.conti@unipg.it`

Abstract. The new trends in the design of race catamarans has introduced new innovations as huge vertical wings instead of main soft sails, and foiling underwater wings. The scope of the paper is the development of a mathematical model of these new features to be implemented in a simulator designed for training purpose. The paper describes the principal assumptions, the simplifications, and the modeling strategies that were adopted in order to obtain a real time simulation. The mathematical model is implemented in an already existing SIMULINK simulator developed at the University of Southampton and exploits its graphical interfaces. The main new feature is the "flying" simulation. The simulator is designed to interact with the in-training team and to feedback the crewmen with realistic cues. Beside training purpose, the simulator could also be a useful tool in comparing different race strategies in order to select the most promising one.

Keywords: Sailing simulator · Crew training · America's cup · Real-time · Simulator · Human interface

1 Introduction

The design and construction of high-speed sailing multihulls is going through a very innovative phase. Since the 2007 America's Cup, with only monohulls, a large number of high performance multihulls have been built. These boats have the power to attract media interest and a larger portion of the general public because of their speed and of the athletic skill required.

Since 2007, one of the most important teams, BMW Oracle, has developed the 90-foot trimaran that won, in 2010, one of the strangest America's Cup ever raced, due to the presence of one catamaran with a classic sail plan, and one trimaran, with a large wing sail. Following that, after the change of the America's Cup rules, a number of AC45 and AC72 class boats have been designed and built. The September 2013 event in San Francisco Bay showed the power of these boats that can be considered as the Formula 1 of the sea (Fig. 1). They are large, beautiful, fast, and built with high-tech materials. They have innovative features such as foils and wings which make them completely new.

The knowledge of how to handle these boats is important not only to win the Cup but also to ensure the safety of the crew. The importance of the latter topic is paramount, as demonstrated by the Artemis AC72 capsize, which led to the loss of life of the Olympic sailor Andy Simpson.

© Springer International Publishing Switzerland 2015
J. Cabri et al. (Eds.): icSPORTS 2014, CCIS 556, pp. 57–70, 2015.
DOI: 10.1007/978-3-319-25249-0_5

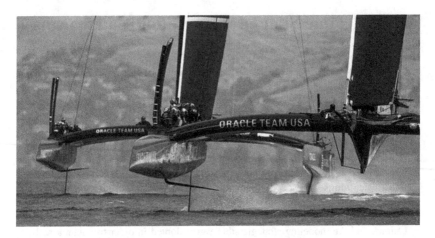

Fig. 1. AC72 Oracle team USA.

These reasons highlight a need for the formulation of sailing simulators, in order to provide the Teams with a key tool. It has to be more realistic as possible and provide a user experience as close as possible to reality in order to allow crew members to train and know how to handle the boat adapting their individual, diverse sailing background to the new boats. These considerations led to the development of an AC45 simulator by University of Southampton students [1]. The scope of this simulator, however, is limited because the mathematical model had only four degrees of freedom, two translations in the plane and two rotations. Due to this, the simulator can simulate with a good reliability only the tack manoeuvre; moreover the sailing in foiling mode is not taken into account. The simulator described in the present paper was formulated using the Southampton simulator as a starting point, and overcomes some of its limitations.

2 The Simulator

The simulator consists of three different parts: the graphical interface, the mathematical modeling and the physical interface.

The graphical interface consists of a screen view of the virtual scene rendering the instantaneous setting of the catamaran. This aspect was touched only marginally in order to verify the reliability of the model which was developed in this work.

The mathematical model of the AC45 provides the boat's response to the different environmental conditions encountered during a race (aero and hydrodynamic forces) as well as to the crew actions. The mathematical model was implemented in a SIMULINK program which is the core of the simulator. In this work only this area is considered.

The physical model aims to provide sailors with a physical reproduction of the catamaran. Using the results of the mathematical model, it is intended to give the crew a more immersive, realistic feel of the boat and of the race scenarios. The physical model is not implemented in the present version of the simulator.

3   Mathematical Modeling

3.1   Geometric Characteristics

The model simulates the behavior of the AC45 catamaran equipped with different appendages in order to make it able to fly over the water (Fig. 2). The main parameters of the AC45 are available in the official America's Cup website but, in order to exactly reply its behavior, some parameters - which are not of public domain - were introduced into the model on the basis of previous experience on catamarans. The main parameters of the boat modeled in the simulator are listed in Table 1. In order to implement new characteristics and to make the simulator able to deal with the new frontiers of technology, the capability to lift over the sea and to "fly" - thanks to the foils- was introduced.

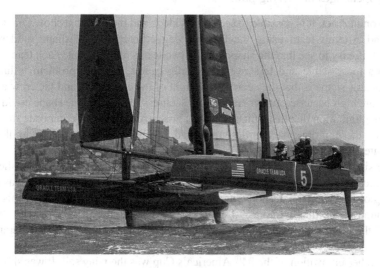

Fig. 2. AC45 Oracle team USA with foils.

Table 1. Main boat parameters.

Geometrical feature	Dimension
Length Overall (LOA)	13.45 m
Bmax	6.77 m
Mast height	21.50 m
Wing width	5.50 m
Upwind sail plane	133 m^2
Downwind sail plane	210 m^2

These new features of the catamaran make it incredibly different from a classical catamaran. When the boat flies, the hull resistance drops to zero and each variation of the rudders position has a big effect on the boat heading. The same sensation could be experienced on fast skiff boats, and this is the reason why many of the team's crewmen came from small dinghies. In this context, the simulator plays an important role on adapting the helmsman and the crew skills to the new boats.

There is a large piece of information in literature about normal catamarans or multihull boats. In fact, they are used to complete the round around the world and to break every year different records because of their speed. But the presence of foils is a new phenomenon, which appeared during the last America's Cup.

Before that date, no team had any experience about it and a massive research effort was carried on to acquire new experience and knowledge. Unfortunately, all the knowledge acquired is proprietary of the teams and held confidential.

3.2   Appendages and Wing Sail

Surfing on internet, it is possible to see some videos and pictures that show Oracle team USA and Artemis team using the L-shape daggerboards and T-shape rudders (see Fig. 1). It is easy to see that the shapes of the two teams are different. Each team tries to reach the most stable and less resistant configuration. Another problem influencing daggerboards shape is that they carry the weight of the entire boat and the crew and the stresses are high because of their small cross section. The appendage shape could suffer also some limitation due the difficulty to obtain sharp angles with composite materials. To solve these problems, the designers had recourse to aerospace technology in composite elements manufacturing.

The simulator model implements a normal daggerboard in order to give the side-force necessary to balance the heeling force. A NACA 0012 horizontal foil was added at its tip of the daggerboard allowing the boat lift. All the characteristics of this shape were found in the literature and 3-D effects were added later [2]. As a result the two parts of the composite daggerboard are considered separately and all the parameters vary independently from each other.

The other innovation of the 34th America's Cup was the wing sail. It was showed to the big public during the America's Cup of 2010, when the Alinghi catamaran lost the Cup versus the big trimaran of Oracle which had a huge wing. The AC45 is characterized by a symmetric wing sail formed by a main wing rotating about the mast and three rear flaps distributed spanwise rotating at 90 % of the chord of the forward wing. Due to the symmetry and the possibility to rotate the four parts, the wing is able to produce lift in both port and starboard tack. The structure of the wing is made of a carbon fiber composite frame covered with a light soft membrane. The crew is able to change during the race the sheeting angle of the main wing, the camber of the whole wing and the twist of the flaps. The advantage of the wing with respect to a classic soft sail is the possibility to produce a larger lift due to absence of turbulence behind the must, yielding a more uniform and continuous pressure on the sail surface [3]. Another important feature is the possibility to have high lift even with low apparent wind angle. That is very important on high speed catamarans; in fact, they can reach a speed twice as large as true wind velocity.

3.3 Reference Systems

In order to represent the motion of the boat, three reference systems are defined (Fig. 3):

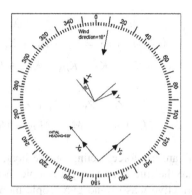

Fig. 3. Water plane representation of the three systems.

- The global world reference system is an absolute reference system independent from time. Healing angles and true wind angles are referred to this system. All the spatial coordinates of the boat are transformed into this reference system and provided to the graphical interface. In Fig. 3 the system is represented by a compass scale.
- The second reference system has the X_0 and Y_0 axes parallel to the water. Considering the initial heading, the X_0-axis corresponds to the centre line and points towards the bow of the catamaran, the Y_0-axis is positive towards starboard, the Z_0-axis is positive downward. The origin of this system is set in the initial position of the centre of gravity of the boat. The corresponding moments are: roll moment M_{xx}, pitch moment M_{yy} and yaw moment M_{zz}. This reference system is defined at the starting time and does not move with the boat; all the integrations are performed in this refrence system.
- The third reference system is solidal with the boat and all the dynamic characteristics are evaluated in this system. It is a right-hand orthogonal system centered on the center of gravity of the boat. At the starting time this reference system is coincident with the X_0-Y_0-Z_0 system.

The forces and moments acting on the AC45 catamaran are calculated at each step during the simulation and these are integrated to obtain the value of the translations and rotations related to the $X_0 Y_0 Z_0$ system. These values are then transformed into the global world system and fed to the graphical interface.

3.4   Dynamic Equilibrium Equations

The simulation model is based on four differential equations as in standard VPP with 4 d.o.f., plus a couple of equations concerning pitch and heave motion (often neglected in standard VPP) which are crucial to simulate a catamaran with lifting foils:

$$
\begin{aligned}
(m + m_x) * \ddot{x} &= X_H + X_{Wi} + X_A + X_{HS} + X_{WS} \\
(m + m_y) * \ddot{y} &= Y_H + Y_{Wi} + Y_A + Y_{HS} + Y_{WS} \\
(I_{xx} + J_{xx}) * \ddot{\vartheta} &= K_H + K_{Wi} + K_A + K_{HS} + K_{WS} + K_{CR} + K_{\dot{\vartheta}} * \dot{\vartheta} \\
(I_{zz} + J_{zz}) * \ddot{\varphi} &= N_H + N_{Wi} + N_A + N_{HS} + N_{WS} \\
(m + m_z) * \ddot{z} &= Z_H + Z_{Wi} + Z_A + Z_{HS} + Z_{WS} + Z_{\dot{z}} * \dot{z} \\
(I_{yy} + J_{yy}) * \ddot{\omega} &= M_H + M_{Wi} + M_A + M_{HS} + M_{WS} + M_{\dot{\omega}} * \dot{\omega}
\end{aligned}
\tag{1}
$$

Where "Xij" and "Yij" are the forces acting on the boat, "Kij" and "Nij" are the moments, "m" and "Iii" are the true mass and gyroscopic moments of the boat while "mi" and "Jii" are the corrective masses and gyroscopic moments introduced to take into account the effects of water interaction with a floating body [4]; the subscripts must be interpreted as follows: HS = Headsail, WS = Wingsail, WI = Windage, A = Appendage, H = Hull, CR = Crew.

With respect to standard VPP, the equations set contains also all the forces in the vertical direction and the pitch moments acting on the boat. The mathematical model does not take into account any coupling effect between the d.o.f. (which, actually, exist but are considered as second order effects) because they should lead to numerical burden and instabilities. Given a set of initial conditions, the differential equations are integrated twice to obtain velocity and displacement for each d.o.f. The integration scheme is based on a fixed step 4th order Runge_Kutta algorithm.

The model changes the setting of the boat according to the actions of the crew. The following parameters are considered: trimming, position of the headsail, position and orientation of the wing and the rudder, twist of the wing, flattening of the headsail. The daggerboards' positions can be modified as they play a basic role on the ability of the crew to complete the manoeuvres. In the present version of the simulator, the crew can change all these parameters during the run using some joysticks and keys on a computer.

The America's Cup showed the importance of fast sailing with the hull lifted above the sea in order to maintain constant high speed. The simulator allows the crew to test all these manoeuvres in an immersive environment, finding the best solution and acquiring the skills to beat the other teams.

The possibility to jibe without touching the water was already known. The new challenge is now to complete also the tack without wetting the hulls. The team that will obtain this result will probably win the Cup. The simulator can offer an interesting tool to improve the catamaran features and the crew skills [5].

With the foil, the problem of the pitch pole is damped but still important in catamarans. When the boat bears away, the bow is pushed into the water and the ability of the crew to set off, first, all the sails and then the headsail, is of fundamental importance. The helmsman as well has to move smoothly the rudder in order to avoid uncontrolled

manoeuvres and preventing the crew members from falling overboard (as happened to Dean Barker in the final race versus Luna Rossa during the Louis Vuitton Cup).

3.5   Forces and Moments

In the sailing boats there are different forces - which are due both to aerodynamic and hydrodynamic components - that make the model complex [6]. Water and air are very well known and there are many references in literature; however, the interaction between them makes the problem more complex and some simplification is required. Moreover, the model has to change depending on the heave of the boat. In fact, if the boat is floating, the hull has a large resistance force arising from the friction resistance, wave resistance, induced resistance and heeling resistance. These components were evaluated with classical formulae as presented on the ORC VPP Documentation [7]. When the boat "flies" these resistances drop dramatically down and the governing forces must be evaluated with different criteria.

The first innovation taken into account in this model is the rigid wing. The forces acting on the wing for any sailing configuration could be evaluated with CFD analyses but this approach is not suitable for a real time simulator due to the heavy and time consuming computations. This difficulty was overcome constructing a three dimensional look up table (LUT) yielding the forces for discrete sets of wing position, true wind speed, and true wind angle. For each discrete parameters' set, the aerodynamic forces have been evaluated with CFD analyses and introduced in the LUT. During the simulation stage, at each step, the simulator enters the parameters values and, though linear interpolation of the data from the LUT, retrieves the aerodynamic forces on the wing.

A second innovation of the new catamarans is the introduction of the foils. They allow the catamaran to heave over the water surface exploiting the more efficient driving force ensured by the innovative wing. In order to take into account their contribution, the hydrodynamic forces acting on the appendages were modeled as follows: the appendages were split in two parts; the first vertical part produces the side force needed to balance the transverse force in order to contrast the leeway drift, the second horizontal part (at the tip of the first parts) is responsible for the vertical forces allowing the heave of the hulls above the sea. These hydrodynamic forces are evaluated through the classical formula:

$$F_{z,} = \frac{1}{2} * \rho * V^2 * C * A \qquad (2)$$

where "V" represents the boat speed and "A" the area of the foils.

The "C" coefficients ("C_l"for lift evaluation and "C_d" for drag evaluation) were calculated (through interpolations) assuming a foil geometry according to the NACA 0012 profile [2]. The real daggerboard has a "V" shape (see Fig. 4A); as the boat starts to lift, the wetted surface becomes smaller and smaller reducing the lift force. In the simulator the daggerboard was modeled as "L-shaped" (Fig. 4B) -in order to simplify the aerodynamic analyses- and its lift force wouldn't change as the boat lifts over the sea. In order to reproduce the true behavior of the real daggerboard, in the model, the area of the horizontal foil is assumed to vary with the lift.

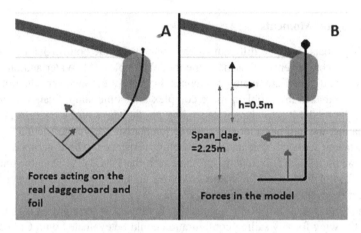

Fig. 4. A- Real daggerboard; B- Modelled daggreboard.

The area is held constant until the boat heave reaches 0.5 m, then the area is linearly reduced reaching a virtual 0 value at 2.25 m (this value is never reached in practice). With this approach, the lift force simulates the real behavior of the foils.

When the catamaran "flies" above the water all the vertical loads are balanced by the foils and the overall equilibrium is ensured by the combination of the forces acting on each foil; the rudder foils are subject to a vertical force directed downwards while the daggerboard foils push the hulls upwards. As the rudders are far from the centre of rotation while the daggeboards are very close, the equilibrium around the Y-Y axis can be ensured with low vertical forces acting on the rudder foils (compared to the forces on the daggerboard foils), for this reason the dagger board foils area is nearly ten times larger than the rudder foils area.

3.6   Cues to the User

In order to ensure efficacy and effectiveness of the simulator, the cues from the simulator to the users are extremely important. The crew must be able to communicate with the simulator and receive the right feedback from it. The torque on the rudder and the wing or the forces from the headsail are very important and allow the sailors to feel the minimum variation of the wind speed, angle of attack and boat speed. Figure 5 summarizes SIMULINK block concerning the heilsail control.

The simulator has three input signals, two sheets positions and one rudder position, and three feedback signals, the torque due to the forces on the sails and the rudder, which are calculated from the computer and send to the joysticks. This means that it is intended for a three members crew. They must work together and interact simultaneously with the simulator. They must synchronously cooperate to keep the boat stable.

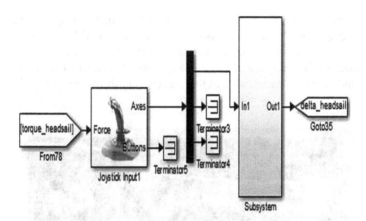

Fig. 5. Headsail input and feedback system.

Even if the simulator does not have a position record yet, the position can be obtained with the supervision of a coach.

The possibility to easily teach the user is the main advantage of the simulators but a second opportunity is represented by the possibility to compare different race strategies and to select the most promising one on the basis of weather forecasting [8].

The crew can also move and change the appendages position. As explained above, the daggerboards position is very important on the manoeuvres. The crew members have the possibility to set the daggerboards in or off as they wish; therefore they can be trained in finding the best settings and the best manoeuvre sequence. In order to check the behavior of the catamaran the crew members can watch through some scope and have the feedback of their actions.

This solution appears very realistic because in the last America's Cup the wear technologies were massively used and all the crew members could check instantly the parameters of their interest.

4 Results

4.1 Switching from Normal Floating Configuration to "Flying" Configuration

The validation of the simulation was performed through a critical evaluation of its results and through some tests. It should be born in mind that a comparison with the results from other simulators is not possible because no other foiling AC45 simulators are available to date (at least to the author's knowledge). The results given below show that the simulator's behavior is in agreement with that of the actual boat. All the main parameters, such as pitch and heave, are consistent with those observed on real boats. As an example, Figs. 6 and 7 display time histories of the main parameters of the boat. In both the figures the time (seconds) is reported on the horizontal axis while in the vertical axis are reported the parameters with their appropriate dimensions (knots for the speed, meters for the heave, degrees for the angles). In Fig. 6 speed, pitch, heave, and heel are displayed. As one can notice, once a speed around 15kts is reached (after 20 s), the catamaran starts foiling and the speed rises dramatically.

The increase of the catamaran speed changes also the apparent wind velocity and apparent wind angle (as expected) and these effects are displayed in Fig. 7.

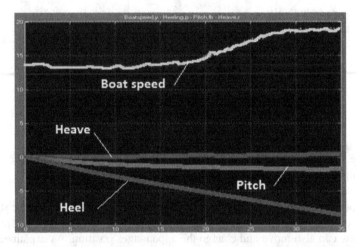

Fig. 6. Time histories of boat main parameters: Boat Speed, Heave, Pitch, Heel.

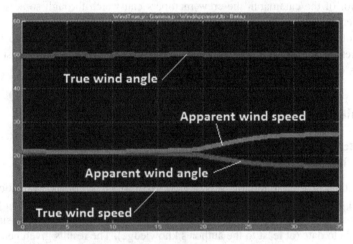

Fig. 7. Time histories of true and apparent wind: True Wind Angle, True Wind Speed, Apparent Wind Angle, Apparent Wind Speed.

4.2 Total Resistance

The graph in Fig. 8 compares the total resistance when the boat sails into water and when it is flying. The graph mustbe read considering that until the boat speed is below 10 kts, the catamaran has all the hull resistance (solid line).

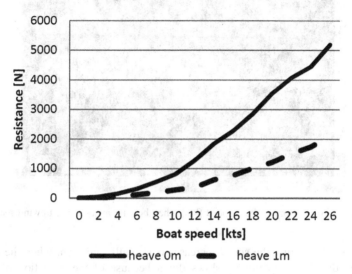

Fig. 8. Resistance[N] vs. boat speed [kts].

Above that speed, the catamaran starts foiling: the hull resistance drops to zero and the appendages' resistance and windage resistance (dashed line) are the only resistance components left.

As soon as the catamaran starts foiling the resistance curve switches from the solid line to the dashed line.

4.3 Bear Away

The behaviour of the simulator with respect to direction changes is important in order to capture the catamaran's motion.

The boat speed on this manoeuvre increases when the helmsman starts to bear away (35th sec.) Fig. 9. It means that the mathematical model predicts correctly the acceleration of the boat when it bears away at the upwind mark. The pitch angle starts to increase and finds a new equilibrium position with the bow closer to the water.

4.4 Luff up

Also in the luff up the results given by the mathematical model are consistent with sailing experience and the expected behavior of a foiling multihull. As displayed in

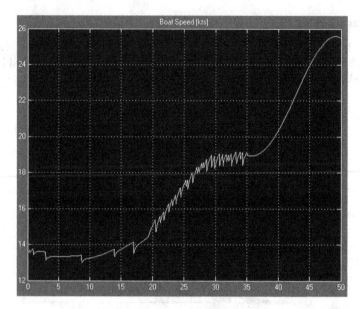

Fig. 9. Time history of boat speed [kts] when bearing away at the upwind mark.

Fig. 10, at the beginning the speed increases marginally and then, when the apparent wind angle drops, the catamaran slows down because of the reduction of the sail forces.

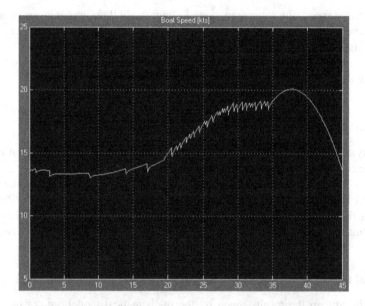

Fig. 10. Time history of boat speed [kts] when luffing up.

5   Graphical Interface

The simulator has a graphical interface to display the boat position and the movements of the boat.

The present implementation is a preliminary version developed at Southampton University [1]. In order to take full advantage of the simulator the graphical interface must be upgraded and more details must be introduced to yield a full immersive environment. Up to now, the existing version is linked with the simulator and gives an essential visual feedback. Figure 11 shows an example frame from the graphical interface.

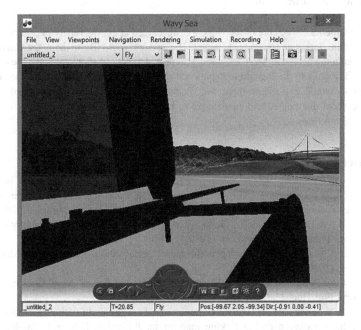

Fig. 11. Example of graphical view.

6   Conclusions and Further Work

The introduction in the simulator of the two new degrees of freedom (pitch and lift) gave the possibility to add the foils to the catamaran. In that way, it was possible to verify the reliability of the mathematical model and it will be possible to provide the in-training crewmen with realistic physical feedbacks. The reproduction of the actual behavior of the real catamaran suggests to complete the project with a physical simulator able to interact with the real users and help the crew to adapt its knowledge to the new boat.

Future modeling work will concern the introduction of the weather conditions (waves and wind) in order to make the simulator able to reproduce all the phenomena.

The improvement of the graphical interface appears fundamental to give the right feeling to the crew. In fact, the graphical interface is the first element of judgment the user may relay on. It can be implemented using waves, splash and more realistic boat details. Finally, a physical model - consisting of a movable platform controlled by the simulator - must be introduced to give a realistic feedback to the crew. The degrees of freedom can be inserted into the physical interface. It will need a movable platform where the movements and the rotations can be implemented. Rudders and sail sheets could be placed in order to provide more realistic environment. They have to be able to givethe user the same forces feeling that the crew experiences in reality, this can be done using some simple actuators. The improvement of the physical interface can follow what is already done with the Formula 1 simulator; this could push the boat simulator towards a new era.

Acknowledgements. The core of the work was developed at the University of Southampton by Filippo Rocchini during an Erasmus exchange. The authors would like to thank the University of Southampton in the person of Mr. Claughton who provided the old simulator and gave new ideas to improve it, thanks to his incredible experience in sailing and in the America's Cup Race.

The authors would also like to thank the Wolfson Unit for the its support; special thanks to Eng. M. Scarponi that helped and encouraged to keep up and to finish the work.

References

1. Breschan, L.M., Lidtker, A., Giovannetti, L.M., Sampson, A., Vitti M.: America's Cup Catamaran Tacking Simulator. Ph.D. Thesis - University of Southampton (2012/2013)
2. Abbott, I.H., von Doenhoff, A.E.: Theory of wing sections: Including a Summary of Airfoil Data. Dover Publications, New York (1959)
3. Haack, N.: C-class catamaran wing performance optimisation. University of Manchester, Manchester (2010/2011)
4. Brennen, C.E.: A Review Of Added Mass and Fluid Inertial Forces. Naval Civil Engineering Laboratory, Port Hueneme (1982)
5. Masuyama, Y., Fukasawa, T.: Tacking simulation of sailing yacht with new model of aero-dynamic force variation during tacking manoeuvre. Journal of Sailing Technology (2011, Article January)
6. Keuning, J.A., Sonnenberg, U.B.: Approximation of the hydrodynamic forces on a sailing yacht based on the delft systematic yacht hull series. Int. HISWA Symp. Yacht Des. Constr., Amsterdam RAI (1998)
7. ORC VPP Documentation 2012. Offshore Racing Congress (n.d.)
8. Scarponi, M., Shenoi, R., Turnock, S., Conti, P.: Interaction between yacht-crew system and racing scenarios combining behavioural model with VPPs. In: 19th International HISWA Symposium on Yacht Design Construction. Amsterdam (2006)

Guiding System for Visually Impaired Running on a Track

Ferdinand Kemeth[1]([envelope]), Sven Hafenecker[1], Ágnes Jakab[2], Máté Varga[2],
Tamás Csielka[2], and Sylvie Couronné[1]

[1] Fraunhofer Institute for Integrated Circuits, Nordostpark 93,
90411 Nuremberg, Germany
{sven.hafenecker,sylvie.couronne,ferdinand.kemeth}@iis.fraunhofer.de
[2] Ateknea Solutions, Tétényi út 84-86, Budapest 1119, Hungary
{agnes.jakab,mate.varga,tamas.csielka}@ateknea.com

Abstract. Sighted people can enjoy many social activities that the visually impaired are denied. Our project has the major goal to develop a
guidance system: A real-time locating system (RTLS) based on radio
signals guides runners with the highest level of safety by estimating the
angle of arrival (AoA) and round-trip time (RTT). First results show the
position accuracy of the proposed locating system with real-world data
with a deviation of less than one metre. Thus we provide an enormous
freedom for the visually impaired runners compared to the other solutions: Blind and sighted runners will have the opportunity to do sport
together without another person's assistance.

Keywords: Real-time locating system · Angle of arrival · Round-trip
time · Visually impaired runners · Guiding system

1 Introduction

In recent years the EU and all its member countries have committed themselves
to creating a barrier-free Europe. There are still many obstacles preventing people with disabilities from fully exercising their fundamental rights including their
Union citizenship rights and restricting their participation in society on an equal
basis compared with non-disabled people. Those rights include the right to free
movement, to choose where and how to live, and to have full access to cultural,
recreational, and sports activities. Regarding sports, particularly running activities, the visually impaired do not have equal opportunities.

The most common way of running is the so-called guided running, in that
blind runners train and race with a sighted runner with the help of a tether [1].
With the Blindtrack project the consortium aims to raise the level of accessibility of the visually impaired to sports, in order to reflect the need for an
effective assistive technology. This would facilitate the well-being of the visually
impaired while decreasing their exclusion from sport and leisure activities. The
proposed system helps visually impaired people to integrate into the community

© Springer International Publishing Switzerland 2015
J. Cabri et al. (Eds.): icSPORTS 2014, CCIS 556, pp. 71–84, 2015.
DOI: 10.1007/978-3-319-25249-0_6

with increasing confidence, better health condition and higher tolerance level of sighted people.

The aim of the Blindtrack project is to develop a running facility embedded in a 400 m athletic track for visually impaired people to run without another person's assistance. Blindtrack will be able to bring significant changes in training opportunities for the visually impaired. The objective is to increase the number of blind and partially sighted athletes with the creation of a tailored infrastructural facility that can be the first step to training without sighted volunteers. Although Blindtrack focuses on visually impaired users, the system provides online available training results to the sighted people: This enhances the market opportunities and further development for small and medium enterprises (SME).

In this article we focus on the project's locating part as follows: Sect. 2 provides an overview for the proposed system and the project organization. Section 3 gives basics on the used locating techniques and Sect. 4 shows the locating performance of the system under development. The last Section summarizes the article together with the next steps [2–6].

2   Blindtrack Overview

The Blindtrack system structure is intended to be built up by three main components:

– the BlackFIR [7] unit which is a high precision locating system,
– the belt unit which is a vibro tactile belt and
– a Central Control Unit (CCU).

The BlackFIR system has the responsibility to locate the athletes on the track in real time, while the belt unit coordinates the athletes with vibrations while running and helps them avoid obstacles and collision situations. The CCU predicts and calculates the different trajectories for each athlete and also filters and singles out the right commands to be sent.

2.1   System Description

Figure 1 shows the general architecture of the complete Blindtrack system. It is necessary to create an own local Blindtrack network on the athletic field, which is completely separated from other public or local area network. This separation ensures that the Blindtrack server is kept safe, prevents the undesired system overloads and shutdowns and makes the operation fast and continuous. The server has a Linux operating system and a runtime environment to fulfil the controlling tasks that includes the calculation of the trajectories, the selection and transfer of the commands. The CCU has also a client side, where one or more computers can connect to the Blindtrack server as client device. The client computer has a graphical user interface (GUI), which helps the operator who is the supervisor of the athletic field and the runners. The GUI is also responsible for the administrative issues and the statistical data display. All these tasks

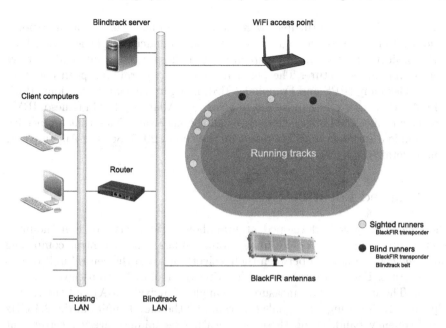

Fig. 1. General system architecture of the Blindtrack.

are not required in real-time conditions, therefore they are detached from the Blindtrack server.

The communication protocol between the modules is based on novel wireless technologies where low latency and high reliability are crucial parameters. The communication with the belt unit will be implemented by Wi-Fi access points that provide easy and fast information transmission, and prevent the interference with the BlackFIR locating system. The belt consists of a driver module and an actuator part. The driver module is responsible for the communication towards the CCU and for the control of the belt actuators. This module also contains a power supply unit, which drives the complete belt and a compass module which determinates the relative orientation of each actuator to the north. The firmware of the belt is responsible for translating the commands relative to north for the actuator. This can minimize the intensity of wireless communication in the Blindtrack system.

BlackFIR is an innovative radio frequency (RF) based locating system, which is able to operate in real time and detects the exact position of each runner on the track. The BlackFIR system consists of several antenna units, mobile transponders carried by athletes and a central unit. The communication between the antenna units and the central unit occurs via Ethernet. The mobile transponder has a special transceiver chip to locate and identify the athletes.

2.2 Project Organization

Blindtrack project management structure was designed and agreed by the consortium members to ensure an effective and straightforward project management mechanism. The main principles were to set up and maintain an organisational structure that ensures the highest technical and financial implementation level of the project, and the efficient exploitation of the project results and effective decision making structure. The partners represent several European countries such as Germany (PPS and Fraunhofer IIS), Hungary (Ateknea Solutions, BSK, INFOALAP), the Netherlands (Elitac), Norway (Adaptor), Spain (Eneso, IBV), and their professional experiences cover all the necessary fields that are needed to conclude a successful project result by the end of 2015. See the Appendix for a more detailed partner description.

3   Adapted Locating System

The BlackFIR system developed at Fraunhofer IIS consists of four mounted receiver units, upto 30 mobile units (transponders) and a central computing unit. The communication between the receiver units and the central unit occurs via Ethernet. For identification and locating the nanoLOC transceiver chip [8] is used. The infrastructure measures the angle of arrival (AoA) and the round-trip time (RTT) using RF signals generated by the mobile units in the 2.4 GHz ISM frequency band. Using these two locating techniques, every receiver unit estimates the direction and distance of the active transponders and sends the results to a central unit, where the position is determined by combining all the available location information.

3.1   Basics of AoA

Adaptive antenna arrays allow estimating the AoA of a received signal [9]. The received signal source has to be in a far field condition. Far field condition results in signal propagation, which is nearly flat. Figure 2 shows the phase alteration on different channels of an antenna array.

In order to estimate the AoA, different high resolution algorithms like Multiple Signal Classification (MUSIC), estimation of signal parameters via rotational invariance techniques (ESPRIT) or the Minimum Variance Capon Beamformer [9] can be applied. These algorithms use the covariance of the different received

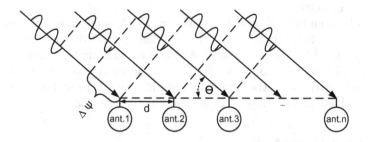

Fig. 2. Received far field signal at the antenna array.

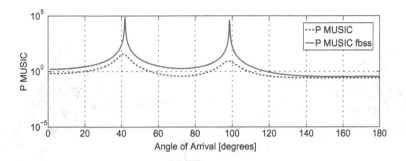

Fig. 3. MUSIC (power) spectrum with and without FBSS.

signals to estimate the AoA. BlackFIR uses a MUSIC algorithm with an additional forward-backward spatial smoothing (FBSS), which improves robustness against multipath by non-line-of-sight (NLOS) signals. The result of the MUSIC algorithm is an angle spectrum, as shown in Fig. 3; position of the maximum of the spectrum show the estimated AoA. The resulting peaks of the MUSIC spectrum get narrower with an additional pre-processed FBSS.

3.2 Basics of RTT

The measurement of distances between a tag ("X") and given receiver positions ("1", "2" and "3") allows the calculation of the tag position, as shown in Fig. 4. BlackFIR uses the nanoLOC transceiver chip to implement the round-trip time (RTT) [10] based distance estimates. The distance is measured by a so called two way ranging procedure. In this procedure time of flight (TOF) is measured by anchor to tag response time and vice versa. This makes it possible to compensate differences in the frequency reference of the tag and the anchor.

Another well-known method to measure distances is to calculate time of arrival (TOA) or time difference of arrival (TDOA). For TOA it is necessary to have synchronisation between the receiver and transmitter, which is often not possible in an adequate way and adequate accuracy. Due to that TDOA is a

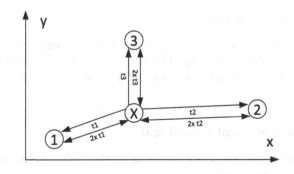

Fig. 4. RTT-based calculation of position.

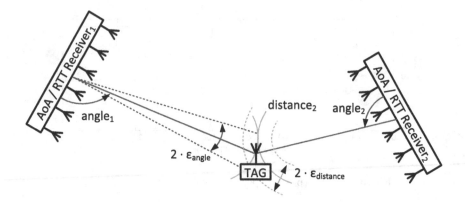

Fig. 5. Principle abstract of BlackFIR RF locating.

possibility, where only the infrastructure is synchronized such as in satellite based global positioning systems (GPS). Using TDOA does not require an extra reply signal which lowers the channel usage and minimizes the measurement time. However RTT requires no synchronisation techniques between the receiver units. Synchronization influences the system infrastructures and increases the cost.

3.3 Infrastructure Setup

The BlackFIR locating system consists of a receiver unit estimating the AoA and the RTT. In order to calculate a two-dimensional position, it is necessary to use at least one of these receiver units. In practice the data is affected by multipath effects, fading and thermal noise based error. In order to improve the estimates, multiple units are used at one scenario in a time duplex sequential measurement procedure as shown in Fig. 5. All available sensor data is collected and combined by a central server were the position is then calculated by either a Kalman filter [11] or particle filter [12] based algorithms.

4   Evaluation

4.1   Measurement Campaign

In order to validate the performance values, a measurement campaign was executed in the Nuremberg stadium. The used test field is a standardised [13] type "A" all-weather running track with eight lanes and a length of 400 m as shown in Fig. 6.

Aim of the Measurement Campaign:

- Identify the performance of the system in the target environment.
- Evaluate the optimal infrastructure structure.
- Optimize the positioning algorithms.

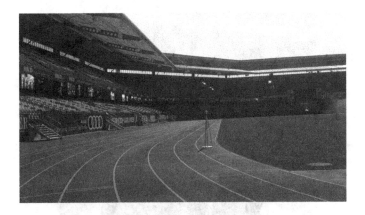

Fig. 6. All-weather running track used for testing.

To analyse the current system performance in different circumstances, the following scenarios were explored:

- **Walking Scenario:** A person was walking along the third running track. The transmitter was affixed at his inner shoulder. The scenario was repeated three times.
- **Running Scenario:** A person was running along the third running track. Like the walking scenario, the transmitter was fixed at his inner shoulder.
- **Scenario with a Bicycle Rider:** A person was riding a bicycle along the third running track.

To get reference information for the positions an optical highly accurate system called iGPS [14] was used. The optical component was mounted on a helmet worn by the athlete as shown in Fig. 7. IGPS ensures point locating accuracy down to 200 µm.

During the different scenarios various datasets of sensor information were recorded to analyse and improve the locating system.

The Types of Raw Information Are:

- In-phase and quadrature components of the RF signal received by the multi-antenna unit for post-processing
- Measured distances between mobile tag and receiver
- Estimated AoA at the receiver units
- Battery life-time information

Four receiver units were placed arround the running track (one unit for every 45-degree bend) in order to ensure line-of-sight to the transponders and for coveraging the whole test field (Fig. 10).

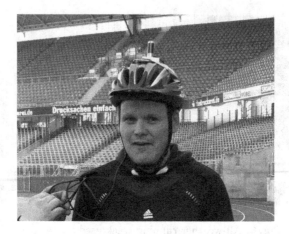

Fig. 7. iGPS probe mounting at the top of a helmet.

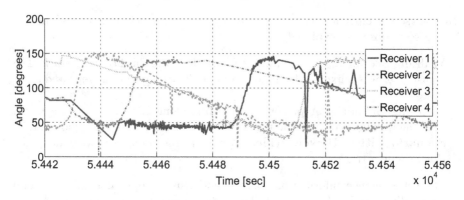

Fig. 8. Angle results based on AoA estimation (Color figure online).

4.2 Analysis

In Figs. 8 and 9 the measured raw AoA and raw distance data over the time are
shown. Each signal of the different receivers is plotted in a different colour.

Every single curve shows spikes depending on channel propagation, fading
and multipath effects (e.g. Receiver 1 in Fig. 8 at $5.451 \cdot 10^4$ s). Because of the
dynamic scenario caused by the runner's movement, these effects can be detected
as outliers and can be compensated later.

Straight lines represent gaps in the information caused by a poor wireless
connection or interferers (e.g. Receiver 4 in Fig. 8 in the time interval between
5.448 and $5.451 \cdot 10^4$ s). However, due to the system's high update rate and
redundancy, it is not necessary to get information from every receiver unit at all
times.

An exemplary view of the actual measured distances and estimated angles is
presented in Fig. 10: Each of the four receiver units show the estimated angle as

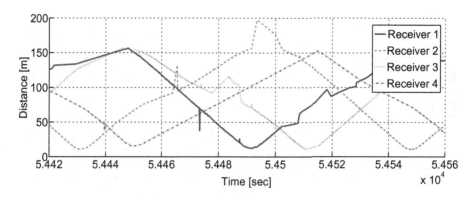

Fig. 9. Distance results based on round-trip time (Color figure online).

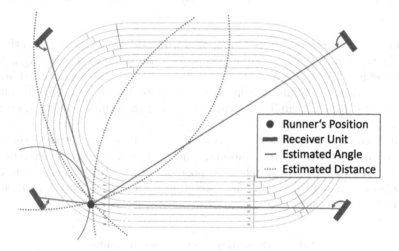

Fig. 10. Position measurement with angle and distance estimation.

a straight line towards the sensor's position. The circles around them represent the measured distances. In best cases, all lines and circles cross in one single point: the athlete's position.

The iGPS reference system was installed in the right part of the stadium due to the need of reference values. The estimated system latency as well as the accuracy of the position is determined by the data observed in that part of the stadium. In contrast to that, the data rate was determined through all data stored in the corresponding scenario.

Figure 11 shows the position trajectory of the measured position values (green line) in the scenario with a running person for two laps. The red line represents the position given by the iGPS reference system which could only cover the right part of the running track. The position estimates have a small variance from the reference position. In addition, the estimates at the right part of the

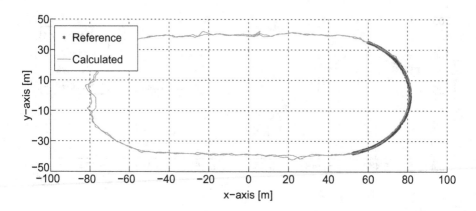

Fig. 11. Measured position in the scenario with a running person (Color figure online).

stadium have better performance compared with position estimates from the left part. The reason is, that the calibration process was performed in the right part, where the iGPS system was installed, so the left antennas were not calibrated as accurate as the antennas on the right of Fig. 10. The measurement results of the two laps are both similiar to each other and explainable by the described effects.

The estimated accuracy of the position is determined by the data that was observed in that part of the stadium, where the iGPS reference system was installed due to the need of reference positions. In contrast to that, the data rate was determined through all data stored in the scenario. Table 1 summarizes the measured system performance.

Table 1. Summary of measurement results.

Estimated latency	440 msec
Data rate	6.6 Hz
Mean deviation	0.689 m
Maximum deviation	2.60 m

"Estimated latency" describes the delay between the athlete's actual and calculated position caused by wireless transmission, network traffic and processing time for the algorithms. "Data rate" describes the update rate of the estimated positions; the update rate for the belt commands sent to the athlete will be less.

The distribution of the measured position errors is shown in Fig. 12.

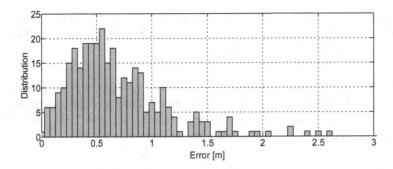

Fig. 12. Distribution of the position error in metres.

5 Summary & Roadmap

In the scope of this article, we presented an adaptation for the BlackFIR locating system to the project needs of Blindtrack. For a system using RTT and AoA technology, we showed detailed results on a measurement campaign and the accuracy of the calculated positions. Our system gives visually impaired people the opportunity to enjoy several social activities with simple installation complexity. Compared to visual tracking systems, we are able to identify and track every runner, even in extreme situations, where the runner is surrounded by many others. In the next steps, adjustments will be made resulting in higher accuracy of the current system and further cost reduction. At the end of this project, the complete system will be tested and evaluated with blind and non-blind runners.

Acknowledgements. The project has received funding from the European Union Seventh Framework Programme (FP7/2007–2013) under the grant agreement No. 605821. It is a 24-month research project that was launched on 1st of January 2014 with the cooperation of nine partners.

Appendix

SME Participants

INFOALAP-Informatics for the Visually Impaired Foundation - Hungary. INFOALAP is actively involved in system specifications, based on its experience with IT for visually impaired, and supports the technology optimization by providing direct evaluation feedback for. They also support hardware and software development by the evaluation of ergonomic aspects by its low vision IT engineers, as well as being active in system tests.

PPS GmbH - Germany. PPS is the supplier of the technology that is capable of real-time detection of the running people in the running track. It closely cooperates with Fraunhofer Institute IIS during the research period and supplies the prototype of the project. PPS defines the prototype in regard of later products and assists the development partners in defining the real use cases as well as the general evaluation of the developments.

ELITAC - Netherlands. Besides supervising, ELITAC's role comes at the phase of tactile belt research and manufacturing. They strongly cooperate with IBV while they are working on the development of the tactile belt. ELITAC has already developed tactile devices but none of them was for the blind.

Eneso Tecnología de Adaptación S.L. - Spain. ENESO is a distributor of BLINDTRACK system. They have a deep knowledge of the accessibility market in Spain, so they will be very active in promoting and placing the system. They will also contribute their experience by testing and validating the product.

ADAPTOR HJELPEMIDLER as - Norway. ADAPTOR plays a significant role in the consortium as the employer of visually impaired and distributor of assistive products and provides the research partners with tangible information on the needs of the market and assist field testing.

RTD Participants

ATEKNEA Solutions Hungary Kft. - Hungary. Ateknea Solutions brings together four research and innovation companies operating at a European level for over 15 years. The group pools the expertise and know-how of more than 130 professionals working in five different locations: Barcelona, Brussels, Budapest, Krakow and Valetta. The innovative companies have successfully participated in more than 150 different projects financed by the European Commission. ATEKNEA is the coordinator of the project and responsible to ensure fluent project flow.

Fraunhofer Institute for Integrated Circuits IIS - Germany. The Institute has a first prototype research result, called RedFIR® know-how and experience that is a state-of-the-art wireless tracking technology that locates people and objects in real time and with high precision. Its main role is to select the best fitting localization technology for a successful project. Compared to current video-based approaches, this radio-based technology offers a major advantage: its tracking capability is not diminished by obstacles obscuring the line of sight. The RedFIR® real-time tracking system is more responsive, accurate and flexible than any comparable technology. Position data is made available in fractions of a second and automatically analysed using pattern recognition and event detection methods. User-specific data preparation and visualization modes are provided in real time. It has an accuracy of a few centimetres, making event detection results and automatically generated statistics highly reliable. In the consortium Fraunhofer will develop a system based on RedFIR® but fulfilling the special needs of visually impaired people and find out a solution that is still affordable and marketable with not forgetting the basic need: maximum accuracy with minimum price.

IBV - Biomechanics Institute of Valencia - Spain. IBV do research to understand the tactile sensing and the perception mechanism in different conditions. Measurements are taken to define the sensitivity of the skin from the density and the intensity point of view as well. They aim to find the optimal sensing positions on the perimeter of the trunk to feel directions with confidence and define the number of the vibrating elements on the belt, and their control to guide a person to the direction we intend to. They have to cooperate closely with Elitac in order to manufacture a defined number of prototypes for testing. A continuous cooperation with the control and communication circuit designer RTD during the control circuit development is also essential.

Other

Budapesti Sportszolgáltató Központ - Hungary. During the project preparation and implementation Budapesti Sportszolgáltató Központ help with practical advices of blind running behaviour and critical points of their secure training. In the testing phase it will make the field available and will actively take part in the validation and dissemination.

References

1. American Foundation for the Blind: Tips for runners with visual impairments (2014). http://www.afb.org/info/living-with-vision-loss/recreation/running-2805/235
2. European Commission: European disability strategy 2010–2020: A renewed commitment to a barrier-free europe (2010). http://eur-lex.europa.eu/LexUriServ/LexUriServ.do?uri=COM:2010:0636:FIN:EN:PDF
3. United Nations: Convention on the rights of persons with disabilities (2007). http://www.un.org/disabilities/default.asp?navid=13&pid=150
4. England Athletics Limited: Running & sprinting with guides (2012). http://metroblindsport.org/downloadlibrary/guide-running-v2.pdf
5. United States Association of Blind Athletes: Sports adaptations (2014). http://usaba.org/index.php/sports/sports-adaptations/
6. Competitor.com: Visually impaired runners ready to tackle boston (2014). http://running.competitor.com/2014/04/news/visually-impaired-runners-ready-tackle-boston_98512
7. Fraunhofer IIS: BLACKFIR 2.4 brochure (2012)
8. Nanotron Technologies GmbH: nanoNET Chirp Based Wireless Networks White Paper (2007)
9. Tuncer, T., Friedlander, B., Yasar, T.: Classical and Modern Direction-of-Arrival Estimation. Academic Press, New York (2009)

10. Std 802.15.4a: IEEE Standard for Information Technology - Telecommunications and Information Exchange Between Systems - LANs and MANs - Specific Requirements - Part 15.4: Wireless MAC and PHY Specifications for LR-WPANs - Amendment 1: Add Alternate PHYs. IEEE Std 802.15.4aTM-2007 edn (2007)
11. Kalman, R.: A new approach to linear filtering and prediction problems. J. Basic Eng. **82**(series d), 35–45 (1960)
12. Arulampalam, M.S., Maskell, S., Neil, G., Clapp, T.: A tutorial on particle filters for online nonlinear/non-gaussian bayesian tracking. IEEE Trans. Signal Process. **50**, 174–188 (2002)
13. DIN 18035–1: Sports grounds - part 1: Outdoor play and athletics areas, planning and dimensions (2003)
14. Metrology, N.: iGPS datasheet: Priciples of operation / Scalebar / i5 Probe kit / Dynamic tracking kit (2010)

Hydrodynamic Resistance Prediction of an Olympic Class Sailing Dinghy Using CFD and Towing Tank Testing

Rickard Lindstrand Levin[1], Christian Finnsgård[2,3](✉), and Jeremy Peter[4]

[1] Division of Marine Design, Department of Shipping and Marine Technology, Chalmers University of Technology, Gothenburg, Sweden
[2] SSPA Sweden AB, Research, Gothenburg, Sweden
christian.finnsgard@chalmers.se
[3] Centre for Sports Technology, Department of Applied Physics, Chalmers University of Technology, Gothenburg, Sweden
[4] Department of Shipping and Marine Technology, Chalmers University of Technology, Gothenburg, Sweden

Abstract. The study presented in this paper aims at investigating, from a hydrodynamic point of view, the most favourable attitude of a sailing dinghy. The procedure includes both an experimental and a numerical approach. Of interest is if these two methods gives analogous results in terms of resistant force and optimal attitude. The numerical study extends to investigating the effects of adding appendages and leeway to the computational model. As this addition strongly affects the computational effort it is also of interest for future reference to see is the same attitude can be predicted this way and thus be discarded from future studies of this kind.

The included verification and validation study reveals that the resistance is greatly under predicted by the numerical method. Furthermore a complete set of results from the numerical predictions was not obtained which makes the goals of the study unfulfilled. This paper also suggest future work on the topic of sailing.

1 Introduction

As a result of the complex three-dimensional shape of the hull, the flow around the dinghy will differ for different attitudes to the direction of motion. This implies the possibility of locating a minimum of hydrodynamic resistance by sailing at a specific angle of trim and heel. Finding the attitude of minimum resistance can potentially increase performance.

Hydrodynamic resistance is not the only effect that must be considered when altering the angle of heel and trim. The projected area for the centerboard and rudder is decreased when the dinghy is heeled, and this is the case for the sail as well. Moreover, stability could be decreased when trimming on the bow. These effects will not, however, be taken into account in this paper. Since the weight

© Springer International Publishing Switzerland 2015
J. Cabri et al. (Eds.): icSPORTS 2014, CCIS 556, pp. 85–106, 2015.
DOI: 10.1007/978-3-319-25249-0_7

of the sailor represents more than half of the displacement, the angles of heel and trim are changed by the position of the sailor.

At professional skill level the competition is very fierce, and thus the element of positioning the sailor can not be neglected. There was no evidence in the studied literature that an investigation of this kind has been conducted before.

The hull used for this study is the Laser dinghy (see www.laserinternational. org for a description), a four-meter-long dinghy crewed by one sailor. The Laser class has been an Olympic discipline since the 1996 Summer Olympics in Atlanta. The class is a strict one-design class, which means that design alterations or additions of any kind are prohibited. Therefore, the manner in which the dinghy is sailed becomes even more important, and any improvements in sailing practice will consequently improve performance in competitive situations at the international level.

The study resulting in the current paper is a part of an initiative at Chalmers University of Technology. The Olympic motto reads; "Citius, Altius, Fortius", which is Latin for; "Faster, Higher, Stronger". These words do not only govern the life of athletes, but many engineers as well. For the last few years Chalmers has supported a project that focuses on the possibilities and challenges for research combined with engineering knowledge on the area of sports. The initiative has generated external funding and has gained great acclaim within Chalmers both among staff and students, in the Swedish sports movement and in the commercial sector. This sports project overall focuses on five sports: swimming, equestrian, floorball, athletics, and sailing.

The paper is composed as follows: Chap. 1 provides the background to the problem and a very brief introduction to the basics of the mechanisms of sailing, the methodology and tow tank test setup. Section 2 presents the computational method. Chapters 4 and 5 recites the verification and Chap. 6 the validation of the simulation results. Chapter 7 finalises the paer with the concluding remarks.

1.1   Background

The governing equations for the dynamics of a fluid are the Navier-Stokes equation (NS) and the continuity equation. However, it is not possible to fully resolve the flow around a ship, yacht or dinghy with these equations ([9], sect. 9.7.1). This is due to the large separation of scales in the domain and the computational effort required to handle it. While the Laser dinghy is four meters long, the smallest scales in the flow, the Kolmogorov scales, are a mere fraction of a millimetre [9]. To resolve of one of the smallest turbulent scales requires approximately four cells in each spatial direction is required. As a result, the resolution of the discretized domain must be incredibly fine in order to fully resolve the flow [5].

For yacht applications, the level of resolution must therefore be limited to that which results in an affordable number of cells. An increase in the cell size leads to a loss of information regarding the smaller turbulent structures. To compensate for this loss of information, turbulence models and near-wall function are introduced to the simulation. Meanwhile, the temporal resolution is neglected all together, as the average quantities of the flow are of greater interest than the instant ones [9]. For example, it may be more valuable to know the average hydrodynamic resistance, rather than the value at each hundredth of a second.

One criterion for neglecting the temporal discretization is that the flow is considered steady, or independent of time. The equations must therefore be adjusted in order to handle averaged quantities. This operation is called Reynolds time averaging, and the new equation is termed the Reynolds time-averaged Navier-Stokes equation (RANS). As the dinghy is assumed to be in flat water in this study, the flow is steady and the RANS equation is used.

1.2 Mechanisms of Sailing

The sail can be understood as a thin wing profile. The wing generates lift and drag, which are defined as the force components that are perpendicular and parallel, respectively, to the apparent wind. The apparent wind is the wind experienced by the sail, i.e. with the boat velocity included (see Fig. 1).

The lift of the sail is the only component acting in the positive direction of motion, and is therefore the only component contributing to propulsion. Furthermore, only one component of the lift is in turn completely aligned with the direction of the yacht. In order for the yacht to move in the right direction, this driving force component must balance the hydrodynamic resistance of the hull, the component of the drag generated by the sail aligned with the opposite direction of the yacht, and the drag generated from the rigging, deck equipment, etc.

The term *leeway* refers to the slight drift of a moving sailing craft toward the leeward side, and is the result of the misalignment of the resultant force of the sail and the direction of motion. This drift is angled in the leeward direction, hence the name leeway. The point at which the pressure field of the sail can be substituted by one force vector is called the center of effort. As the center of effort is dependent on the pressure distribution, it is not trivial to identify, though its location can be estimated at the sails surface center. As the center of effort of the sail is not at the same height as the center of pressure for the hull and keel, a heeling moment will also be generated, resulting in the heel angle.

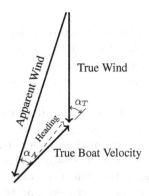

Fig. 1. Working wind speeds and directions. The leeway is the difference between the heading and the true boat velocity.

1.3   Methodology

Prior to the investigation of heel and trim variations, a verification and validation study (v&v) will be performed. This study will be conducted in order to identify the amount of error to be expected from the simulations, and consequently, their relative trustworthiness. Section 3 will further explain the verification procedure.

1.4   Towing Tank Test Setup

Preparing the dinghy for tow tank testing necessitated modifications. An aluminium frame was fitted to the deck around the cockpit. This frame provided a point at which to attach the towing device and also served to accommodate the weights used to position the dinghy in the desired attitude. The appendages were also removed in order to facilitate what will be called a bare hull case. The final modification consisted of the addition of points at which to attach string connected to the measuring devices used to accurately measure heel and trim during speed tests. Figures 2 & 3 display the test frame on the deck.

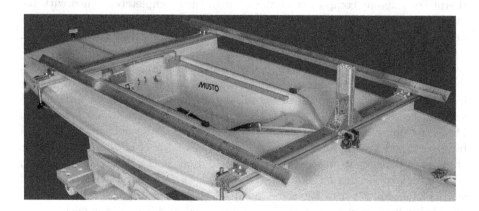

Fig. 2. Towing attachment and weight racks on deck.

The towing device is attached to the top of the vertical aluminium profile. As the towing force is not applied through the center point of the hydrodynamic resistance, a trimming moment is hereby introduced. This moment will not be similar to an actual sailing case, as the towing point does not coincide with the center of effort.

The arm of the towing devise was set up so as to be horizontal for the static cases. This meant that at higher speeds when the dinghy meets with a considerable draft change, the arm would no longer be horizontal, and the towing force would pull the dinghy slightly downward. This would create an increase in displacement, which would in turn affect resistance. Thus, the simulations to be performed could not be set to free sinkage and trim. Due to limited testing time, the heel tests were only performed as heel to starboard tests.

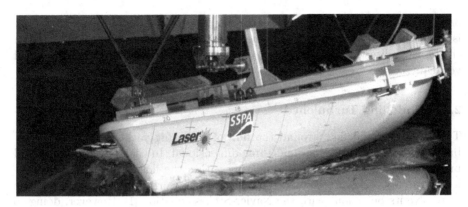

Fig. 3. Test setup during a run, loaded to an heel angle.

The brackets that help hold the frame in place are located on the railing of the dinghy, as illustrated in Fig. 2. As the heel angle increased, the starboard side brackets began interfering with the spray from the bow wave. They were therefore removed from that side and from these tests were rerun.

During the test runs, a bailing pump was added on the flooring of the cockpit to guard against excess water. This excess water was a product of the not completely watertight self-bailer device, which was given to leak by the reversal of the test setup back to the starting position in the towing tank after each run.

2   Computational Method

2.1   Governining Equations

The equations that govern fluid flow are derived from basic physical principles and described by the mathematical statements of the conservation laws of physics: the conservation of mass and momentum. The Navier-Stokes equations are derived from the conservation laws and from several underlying assumptions, and are used to predict the resistance forces that result from pressure and viscosity.

Basic Assumptions. The Navier-Stokes equations are based on the assumptions that the fluid is a continuum, that is, a continuous substance, as opposed to an aggregate of discrete particles. In the case of water, the flow is commonly considered incompressible, rendering constant the density ρ and the viscosity μ. The Navier-stokes equation is then time averaged in order to arrive at the RANS equation

Coordinate System. The simulations are not set up to account for changes in sinkage or trim, as a result of the unnatural trimming moment and the vertical force component created by the towing device. The simulation is also assumed to be steady, that is, it is assumed the dinghy will not move relative to waves or in time. In the global Cartesian coordinate system employed here, the origin is at the bow on the centerline at the undisturbed water level, x is directed in the forward direction of the dinghy, y is directed to starboard and z is directed vertically.

2.2   Modelling Turbulence

Typically, the fluid flow around the hull of a moving yacht is turbulent. Turbulence is irregular, random and three-dimensional. In such flows, velocity and pressure fluctuates continuously, creating within the flow a spectrum of turbulent structures. Despite the irregular nature of a turbulent flow, it is possible to resolve its behaviour with the Navier-Stokes equation [1]. However, doing so requires that the spatial and temporal discretizations are capable of capturing all scales in the flow. This is not possible for ship applications, as the smallest scales are minuscule in relation to the length of the hull, and this in turn leads to unreasonable computational effort.

Therefore the RANS equations are used instead. Time averaging means dividing the instant properties into a mean and a fluctuating part:

$$u_i = \bar{U}_i + u_i'$$
$$P = \bar{P} + p' \tag{1}$$

Insertion of the decomposed terms from (1) into the Navier-Stokes equations gives rise to the Reynolds-averaged Navier-Stokes (RANS) equations. The expression of the incompressible Newtonian fluid in the Einstein notation is:

$$\frac{\partial \bar{U}_i}{\partial t} + \frac{\partial \bar{U}_i \bar{U}_j}{\partial x_j} = -\frac{1}{\rho}\frac{\partial \bar{P}}{\partial x_i} + \frac{\partial}{\partial x_j}\left[\nu\left(\frac{\partial \bar{U}_i}{\partial x_j} + \frac{\partial \bar{U}_j}{\partial x_i}\right) - \overline{u_i' u_j'}\right] \tag{2}$$

In the Eq. 2 the term $\overline{u_i' u_j'}$ appears from the fluctuating values. Known as the Reynolds Stress tensor, this term is an unknown. In order to close the equation system and solve for all the unknowns, the Reynolds stress tensor must be modelled. This is commonly termed the closure problem. The physical interpretation of this term is the influence of turbulence. To account for this unknown term a turbulence model is used.

There are various ways to model the Reynolds stress tensor, including the use of algebraic models, one-equation models, two-equation models, algebraic stress models and Reynolds Stress models. Each of these turbulence models varies in terms of computational requirements and accuracy.

Two turbulence models were implemented in the software: the two-equation Menters Shear Stress Transport model (SST $k - \omega$) and the explicit algebraic stress model (EASM). A description of these models is available below.

Menters SST $k - \omega$ Model. Menter proposed the SST $k - \omega$ model in 1992 in order to improve the performance of the near-wall turbulence modelling of the commonly used two-equation $k - \omega$-model [11]. The SST $k - \omega$ model uses the turbulent kinetic energy k, the turbulence frequency $\omega = \epsilon/k$ (dimension: s^{-1})

and the Boussinesq assumption to compute the Reynolds stresses. The Boussinesq assumption is the presumed relation linking the Reynolds stress tensor to the velocity gradients and the turbulent viscosity. When a turbulence model uses the Boussinesq assumption, it then qualifies as a 'linear eddy viscosity model'. This two-equation turbulence model uses one modelled transport equation for each of the two variables, k and ω. The *omega*-equation is derived from the ϵ-equation in the $k - \epsilon$-model by simply substituting the relation $\epsilon = k\omega$. Though these equations are not displayed here in detail, it is nevertheless important to understand the manner in which these transport equations are constructed. For both equations, the structure is as follows [17]:

$$
\begin{aligned}
\text{Rate of change of } k \text{ or } \omega \;+\; & \text{Transport of } k \text{ or } \omega \;= \\
\text{Transport of } k \text{ or } \omega \text{ by } & \text{turbulent diffusion} \\
+\; & \text{Rate of production of } k \text{ or } \omega \\
-\; & \text{Rate of dissipation of } k \text{ or } \omega
\end{aligned}
\tag{3}
$$

The SST $k - \omega$ model combines the benefits of the Wilcox's $k - \omega$ model at the near-wall and the performance at the freestream and shear layers of the $k - \epsilon$ model. This is why Menters SST $k - \omega$ model is suitable for a wide range of CFD applications [15]. Additionally, assessments of this turbulence model have suggested that it offers superior performance in the case of an adverse pressure gradient boundary layer [17]. An adverse pressure gradient leads to lower kinetic energy of the fluid, and hence to a reduction of its velocity. If the pressure increase is large enough, the fluid direction can be reversed; this is what occurs in flow separation, a phenomenon that typically occurs at the transom of a boat like the Laser. Therefore, this turbulence model seems to be well suited for the current CFD application.

EAS Model. The Explicit Algebraic Stress Model (EASM) proposed in Wallin and Johansson [18] provides an alternative to linear eddy viscosity models (such as the SST $k - \omega$) based on the Boussinesq assumption. Often, linear eddy viscosity models fail to offer satisfactory predictions for complex three-dimensional flows. This leads to nonlinear stress-strain relations that contradict the Boussinesq assumption [6]. Nevertheless, owing to their high level of stability, these linear eddy viscosity models are commonly used in the industry [17].

The original algebraic stress model (ASM) model is not often used as a result of robustness issues and frequent instances of singular behaviour [2]. Both of these issues are addressed in the EAS Model by suggesting treatment of the non-linear term by the production-to-dissipation rate ratio, and the number of tensor bases used to represent the explicit solution of those equations.

2.3 The Volume of Fluid Method (VOF)

The VOF method is a multiphase flow method that computes the interaction of several fluids or phases of a fluid present in the same domain, and obtains the interface between these fluids [10]. For the purposes of yachting applications, implementation of this method allows for the accurate inclusion of the computation of the water surface elevation around the hull.

The VOF method calls for the solving of the same RANS equation as for single-phase flows. The difference lies in a phase indicating function γ [7]. This phase, also called the colour function or volume fraction, displays the measure of the mixture of phases in each cell. For instance, if $\gamma = 1$, the cell is completely occupied by phase one, and if $\gamma = 0.3$, 30 % of phase one and 70 % of phase two are present in the cell. In terms of yachting applications, the two present fluids are water and air. As air is included in this method, the spatial discretization must extend above the waterline as well. This does, of course, increase the computational effort of the simulation, but it offers a significantly more accurate physical representation of the waves, as will be explained below.

The physical fluid properties used in the RANS equation for a multiphase flow are a blend of the properties of the present fluids. The computational properties are blended in the following manner:

$$\rho = \rho_w\gamma + \rho_a(1 - \gamma) \qquad\qquad \mu = \mu_w\gamma + \mu_a(1 - \gamma) \qquad (4)$$

To track the motion of the interface a separate transport equation for the color function is used:

$$0 = \frac{\partial\gamma}{\partial t} + v_i\frac{\partial\gamma}{\partial x_i} \qquad (5)$$

This method does, however, give rise to a numerical problem regarding the smearing of boundaries between the phases over several cells. This smearing denotes that the water surface is constituted by a gradual change in density between water and air. As the water surface is a discontinuity, a jump in density, this smearing represents an unwanted phenomenon. It is a result of the convective averaging being conducted across the water surface. The remedy for this smearing is to implement, in the code, a way to detect the presence of a boundary [8] and treat the bounded areas separately. In the Shipflow software, the smearing problem is addressed by implementation of a compressive discretization scheme, as suggested by [12].

To render visible the surface of the water, the distribution of the colour function is evaluated. Where $0 < \gamma < 1$ there is a mixture between the fluids and the free water surface is found. As mentioned, however, the boundary between the phases may be smeared, and therefore a specific value of γ is selected to display the surface.

The VOF method belongs to the class of surface capturing methods. In such methods, the interface between two fluids is computed somewhere inside the domain. The main difference from single-phase surface tracking methods is that, in this case, the dynamics of the air are also computed. In single-phase methods, the water surface geometry forms the top boundary of the domain, and thus these methods do not take the air into account. The geometry of the top of the domain is then in every time step or iteration updated according to the kinematic and dynamic free surface conditions, and a new grid with new top geometry is generated for the next iteration [9]. In the VOF method, the free surface conditions are automatically satisfied. Furthermore, surface capturing methods have the advantage of being able to capture overturning waves, drops and complex surface features.

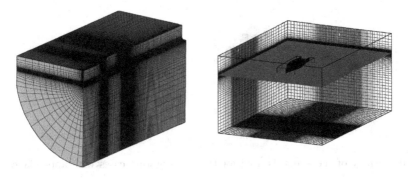

Fig. 4. H-O-grid for the symmetric cases used during the V&V, and boxed grid used for the investigation.

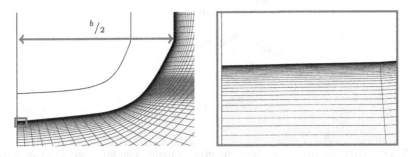

Fig. 5. Display of the cell density near the walled boundary of the hull. $y_1^+ \approx 1$.

For the purposes of this paper, the advantages of the VOF method in the form of physical representation outweigh the disadvantages of computational cost and numerical instability, and the VOF method will therefore be used for all resistance computations.

2.4 Numerical Representation

A structured H-O-grid defines the domain around the hull. This grid layout is desirable because it will generate cells that are roughly aligned with the direction of the flow and fitted to the geometry. Three different structured grids the H-O-grid, H-H-grid and O-O-grid are used to cover each part of the domain. The grid type refers to the shape of the overall domain. The first two grid layouts are displayed in Fig. 5, respectively. The dome-shaped O-O-grid, used around the appendages, is illustrated by Fig. 4.

The near-wall cells must be thin to allow for representation of the velocity profile in the viscous sublayer of the boundary layer, as the gradient of the velocity profile defines the amount of viscous resistance. Thus no wall functions were used. The near-wall cells distribution can be observed in Fig. 6.

The H-O-grid layout is used, as displayed in Fig. 4, only in the verification and validation phase, as the hull is then oriented straight against the flow,

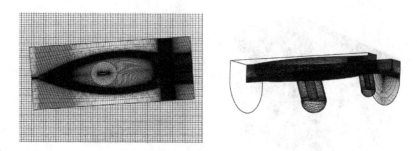

Fig. 6. Display of the subgrids used for the investigation cases with appendages and leeway.

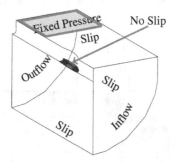

Fig. 7. Boundary conditions for the symmetric domain. The same boundary definition is valid for the boxed grid.

which means that the case is symmetric. In these cases, the simulations are also symmetric along the centerline. The H-H-grid, also called box, is used as the main structure for the simulations of the heel and trim variations. Figure 4 demonstrates this grid layout. The geometrical representation of the hull and appendages was then added to the domain in the form of overset component grids. When these component grids were added, they were also given the selected angles of heel and trim corresponding to the ones obtained at speed during the towing tank tests.

The boundary conditions for the domain are displayed in the following Fig. 7. The slip boundary condition is in practice the same as symmetric, which is why the symmetry boundary is also marked slip. The space above and behind the dinghy is also discretized in two separate grid blocks which are removed from the figure for better visibility.

3   Verification Method

As the governing equations are implemented in a computer code, the fields of the flow properties must be discretized into smaller fluid cells to which the equations are then applied. The differential equations must be linearized and discretization schemes must be applied in order to estimate derivatives and face values.

The size of the cells in the domain impacts the flows representation. In general, the smaller the cells, or the larger the amount of cells in the domain, the better the representation of the flow field [17]. The number of cells will influence to a great degree how computationally demanding the simulation will be.

The flow properties are stored in the center of each cell. The cells interact, however, by way of their adjoining faces, which means that the quantities must be interpolated to the boundary from the centers. This is done according to an interpolation scheme implemented in the code. To determine how well the interpolation scheme is performing in terms of numerical accuracy, a Taylor expansion of a convective term (a derivative) is conducted [17]. When the low order terms are cancelled, the one left with the lowest degree of dependency on the cell size defines the scheme's order of accuracy. The higher order terms in the Taylor series are neglected and the sum is truncated so as to only contain the one defining term.

However, the theoretical order of accuracy, or the decrease in error, might not be observed when refining the grid. This may be attributable to the fact that the refinement of the grid is not completely uniform, to the fact that the wall distance necessary for a turbulence model to be activated is not scaled correctly, or to the fact that the aspect ratio of the cells changes. One further explanation for the inability to obtain the theoretical order of accuracy is that the truncated higher order terms in the Taylor expansion are in fact important for representing the behaviour of the decrease in error.

Any difference between the real flow case and the simulated case in any given quantity is called an error. These errors can be subdivided into two categories: physical modelling errors and numerical modelling errors. Physical modelling errors originate from a faulty model of the physical phenomena at hand, for example, the use of inadequate equations to describe the current phenomena. By contrast, numerical modelling errors derive from the procedures used to solve the equations in the computer. Such errors might include the incorrect rounding off of numbers, incomplete convergence, insufficient spatial discretization, or a diffusive discretization scheme [9].

To ensure the trustworthiness of the CFD simulation, the expected error must be quantified [14]. Here the quantification of the major numerical modelling error; the spatial discretization error, will be explained. The other numerical modelling errors are considered small in comparison and excluded from the verification study; this is possible if the grid refinement factor r is greater than 1.1 [16]. In a pure validation study, the results of the simulation are compared to the data from tests, making the physical errors and the modelling errors indistinguishable.

The verification procedure, called a grid dependence study, aims to observe how a chosen variable, called S, changes according to change in the spatial discretization. In this study, the total resistance force of the dinghy is used. The resistance force will then be plotted as a function of the cell size h for each grid refinement. The data points collected from the simulations of the different grids will then be curve fitted to a certain function and extrapolated to display a hypothetical zero cell-size case.

Furthermore, the verification study also offers an accurate view of which errors can be expected as computational effort inevitably increases and the grid becomes more refined. The method for extrapolation consists of an application of the generalized Richardson extrapolation, called least square root method (LSR).

3.1   Richardson Extrapolation

The equation for the Richardson extrapolation is:

$$S_i = S_0 + \alpha h_i^{p_o} \tag{6}$$

The three unknowns require three solutions, or results from the use of three different grids. The three solutions form a nonlinear system of equations that have an analytic solution [14] in which r denotes the constant grid refinement factor $r = {h_{i+1}}/{h_i}$ and $\varepsilon_{ij} = S_i - S_j$:

$$p_o = \frac{\ln \frac{\varepsilon_{32}}{\varepsilon_{21}}}{\ln r} \tag{7}$$

$$\alpha = \frac{\varepsilon_{21}}{r^{p_o} - 1} \tag{8}$$

$$S_0 = S_1 - \frac{\varepsilon_{21}}{r^{p_o} - 1} \tag{9}$$

3.2   The LSR Method

The drawback of the Richardson interpolation is that it can only be used when the solutions are in the asymptotic range of convergence, which means that the cell size must be sufficiently small so as to render the higher order terms insignificant (this criterion can be quantified in two ways [13]). This in turn requires that the grids are very fine in order to achieve the asymptotic range [4]. The large computational effort required for this made the LSR method more unsuitable for this study (the method for dealing with the scatter of grids considered too coarse for the explained method is proposed in by Eca and Hoekstra, [4]). The three coefficients to Eq. 6 are then found by minimizing the following expression:

$$f(S_0, \alpha, p_o) = \sqrt{\sum_{i=1}^{ng} (S_i - (S_0 + \alpha h_i^{p_o}))^2} \tag{10}$$

Where ng is the number of grids used. When using this method, more than three grids are required in order to account for the scatter. This study used seven grids.

3.3   Uncertainty

As the Navier-Stokes equations are not directly solved, numerical models are applied to the simulation. In doing so, not only is the error based on the difference with respect to the test results of interest, but the uncertainty of the simulation itself [19]. This uncertainty refers to the interval in which the exact solution is expected to be found.

The purpose of the LSR method is to include the exact solution within the error band with 95 % confidence [3]. This method, which is an empirical one, is made and adjusted to fit the test results presented at the workshop of Eca and Hoekstra [3] in a paper of theirs [4]. The computation of uncertainty with the LSR method is governed by the observed order of accuracy p_o, in the following manner:

1. If $p_o > 0$:

$$0.95 \leq p_o \leq 2.05 : U_{sn} = 1.25\delta_{RE} + U_{sd} \tag{11}$$

$$p_o \leq 0.95 : U_{sn} = min\left(1.25\delta_{RE} + U_{sd},\ 3\delta_{RE}^{12} + U_{sd}^{12}\right) \tag{12}$$

$$p_o \geq 2.05 : U_{sn} = max\left(1.25\delta_{RE} + U_{sd},\ 3\delta_{RE}^{02} + U_{sd}^{02}\right) \tag{13}$$

2. If $p_o \leq 0$ and $\sum_{i=2}^{n_g-1} n_i \geq INT\left(n_g/3\right)$, where $n_i = 1$ if $(S_{i+1} - S_i)(S_i - S_{i-1}) < 0$:

$$U_{sn} = 3\delta_{\Delta M} \tag{14}$$

3. Else :

$$U_{sn} = min\left(3\delta_{\Delta M},\ 3\delta_{RE}^{12} + U_{sd}^{12}\right) \tag{15}$$

Where:

– the δ_{RE}^{02} and the δ_{RE}^{12} are obtained from curve fitting the following functions in the same manner as described above in Sect. 3.2

$$\delta_{RE}^{02} = S_i - S_0 = \alpha_{02}h_i^2 \tag{16}$$

$$\delta_{RE}^{12} = S_i - S_0 = \alpha_{11}h_i + \alpha_{12}h_i^2 \tag{17}$$

– the $\delta_{\Delta M}$:

$$\delta_{\Delta M} = \frac{\Delta_M}{\left(h_{n_g}/h_1\right) - 1} \tag{18}$$

where the Δ_M is the maximum data range, $max\left(|S_i - S_j|\right)$.
– the U_{sd}, U_{sd}^{02} and U_{sd}^{12} are the standard deviations of the curve fitted functions: 6, 16 and 17. For example for Eq. 17, the standard deviation is found by minimizing the following expression:

$$U_{sd} = \sqrt{\frac{\sum_{i=1}^{ng} \left[S_i - (S_0 + \alpha_{11}h_i + \alpha_{12}h_i^2)\right]^2}{n_g - 3}} \tag{19}$$

4   Systematic Variation of Numerical Parameters

4.1   Numerical Parameter Study

From the first simulations of this study the resistance was predicted to $\sim 7\%$ below the test data, which was not satisfactory. In order to figure out how to improve the result, the parameters of fluid density ratio, height of domain, turbulence models and local grid refinement were systematically investigated. The outcome of these studies will be presented in this section.

Fluid Density Ratio. This investigation was considered valuable for this study as the default density ratio in the software was set to a non-physical value. The motivation for using a non-physical value was that the simulations become more numerically stable for values closer to one, which means two fluids of the same properties. The result of this investigation can be seen in the following figure:

Notice in Fig. 8 that the trend is diverging as the density ratio decreases and goes toward a value of the physical density ratio of 0.0013. No results from values below 0.0013 are reported because these simulations did not converge.

The difference of 0.90 % decrease from 0.0013 to 0.01 is not considered insignificant. However, as the results in the region of low density ratio are diverging rapidly, these results are not trustworthy and this quantification shall be viewed with caution.

Domain Height. This investigation was done in order to see the effect of the height of the domain on the resistance but also the free water surface geometry in the transom area. Water on the transom was appearing in the simulations even though the transom evidently was clear during the towing tank tests. The height of the domain here refers to the height of the volume above the water

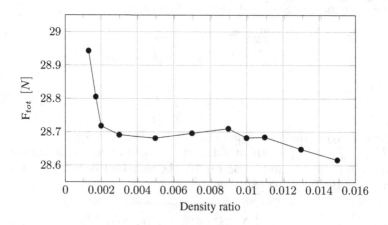

Fig. 8. Result of density ratio investigation. The default value in Shipflow was set to 0.01. The percental difference from 0.0013 to 0.01 is 0.90 % decrease.

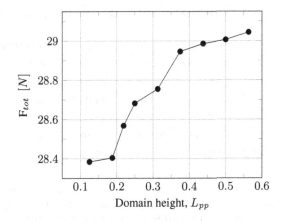

Fig. 9. Result of domain height investigation, domain height refers to the height above the static water surface. Default value in Shipflow was set to 0.5.

surface, occupied by air. The number of cells in the z direction was kept constant when the domain height was changed. The results of this investigation can be seen in the following figure:

Notice in Fig. 9 that the resulting force increases rapidly until 0.375 Lpp. The result from the investigation shows a decrease by 2.27 % from 0.563 to 0.125, with a plateau starting 0.375 Lpp. Domain heights over 0.563 Lpp gave diverging simulations.

Turbulence Model. The selected software Shipflow implements two turbulence models: SST $k - \omega$ and EASM, see Sect. 2.2. As the different turbulence models give good results for different types of flows, both of these were tested in the validation case. The results are presented in Table 1. Concluded from this investigation is that the SST $k - \omega$ model is the superior one for this case. The EASM did not only predict a too-low total resistance, it also took a lot longer to converge. The medium-density grid with the EASM converged with an oscillating trend, and a mean value over 2000 iterations had to be selected. This interval represented roughly two periods of the oscillating behaviour. The SST $k - \omega$ was then used for the forthcoming simulations.

Transom Area Cell Density. His investigation also originated in having water creeping up on the vertical transom of the dinghy. The cause of this water was thought to be an insufficient resolution of the grid at the corner where the transom meets the bottom of the hull.

A consequence of refining the grid locally in the transom area is the grid density at midships. Stretching functions are used in the meshing tool of the software, which makes the very fine cells gradually grow larger with a certain factor. This makes the cells at midships rather large as a limited number of cells is used to cover the length between perpendiculars. This could have been avoided

Table 1. Result of the turbulence model investigation for three different grids.

# cells, M	Turb. mod.	A_w, $[m^2]$	F_{tot} [N]	Difference
4.9	$kw - SST$	3.155	29.00	−6.8 %
4.9	EASM	3.168	27.05	−13.0 %
5.4	$kw - SST$	3.155	29.04	−6.6 %
5.4	EASM	3.170	26.64	−14.3 %
6.4	$kw - SST$	3.154	29.10	−6.44 %
6.4	EASM	3.173	26.57	−14.6 %

Table 2. Result of the transom grid refinement investigation. The cell density is in the lonitudinal direction, in the region aft of the transom. (To save computational effort the region of refinement is concentrated in the last case, which is why the cell count is still 8.9 million).

Density, L_{pp}^{-1}	# cells, M	F_{tot}, [N]	Difference
600	4.7	28.84	−7.14 %
3'600	5.9	29.08	−6.50 %
7'500	8.9	29.09	−6.46 %
30'000	8.9	29.03	−6.65 %

by adding more cells in this area, but as the transom was the area of interest in this investigation this was not done. The longitudinal direction was selected for refinement. The results of this investigation can be seen in Table 2.

The conclusion of the grid refinement was that the transom water could be reduced by refining the transom grid, but it could not be totally cleared. However, the sought gain in resistance was almost negligible and the cost for resolving the flow was significantly increased. This concluded that the transom grid was not the major cause of the too-low predicted total resistance.

4.2   Result of the Verification Study

After selecting the best settings from the numerical parameter studies, the following verification was obtained; (as shown in Fig. 10).

Evident in this grid-dependence study is that there is a strong grid dependency. This means that a substantial increase in grid definition should be able to eliminate the ∼ 7 % error. The problem associated with a further increase is the lack of memory on the machines used to run the simulation during this study. The limit for the available 24 GB seemed to be around 14.5 million cells.

A further refinement of r equal to the 4th root of 2 would result in ∼ 20.3 million cells, but a higher refinement factor is probably needed as there is no improvement observed for the finest presented grid. The conclusion of the grid dependence study is that the grid setup from grid 2 shall be used. To decide

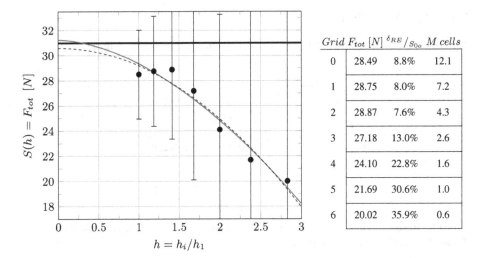

Fig. 10. *Even keel 4 kts.* Test data $= 31.1$ N; $S_{0a} = 30.59$; $S_{0o} = 31.24$; $p_a = 2$; $p_o = 1.75$. Where subscript a and o means analytic and obtained respectively. ___ = Towing tank test; ___ = Obtained convergence; ___ = Analytic convergence.

which grid refinement results in a reasonable error, the result is weighed against the computation time. As grid 2 gave the best results and did not have the highest computation time, it was selected.

Grid dependency for an appendage and leeway case was not done, as the grid settings for the boxed grid, required to include leeway, were not successfully changed. This was due to lack of knowledge in the meshing tool, which led to an inability to systematically refine the grid.

5   Validation Results and Discussion

The main investigation of the paper was to see if the minima in resistance could be predicted at the same angles of heel and trim, using the following methods: bare-hull towing tank tests, bare-hull simulations and simulations with appendages and leeway. If this is the case, the more time-consuming asymmetrical simulations needed for handling the leeway can be rejected for future investigations of this kind. The leeway simulations with the appendages are interesting because they represent real sailing conditions in the most accurate way possible in a steady state setup.

The cases that are included in this study are heel variation for zero trim and the trim variation for zero heel. To find a global minima in resistance combinations of heel and trim have to be simulated as well. A full series of simulations of heel and trim variation was not completed. This was thought to be due to a lack of knowledge in the software, that it is still a young application of the VOF method and that it is usually handles ships of a very different kind. The results of the simulations that are finished are shown in the following section.

5.1   Heel Variation

The results of the systematic heel variations are presented in Fig. 11.

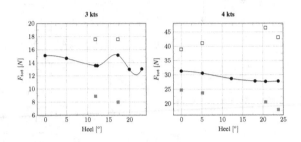

Fig. 11. Result of heel variation. ● = Test data; ■ = Bare hull simulations; □ = Appendage and leeway simulations.

The bare-hull simulations that are finished, and shall be validated against the towing tank test data, are still predicting very low resistance. This is despite the use of the selected numerical parameters from the variation study.

Concluded from the available results from the four-knots-heel variation for the bare-hull cases is that the error is larger than the error obtained in the verification study. The best grid density was then found to be one containing 4.3 million cells and the settings for this grid would now be used for all the simulations during the investigation. The exact grid settings, however, could not be used, as the grid layout will be changed. The grid layout used in the verification study was H-O-grids, explained in Sect. 3.1. For the investigation part, however, the boxed and overlapping grid was used. The reason for this was that the simulations including leeway could not be done in the H-O-grid. The bare-hull simulations were also computed using the boxed grid during the investigation to eliminate the effect of different grid types on a comparison.

The setup of the boxed grid with the selected settings was not done success-fully. The reason for this was a lack of knowledge in the meshing tool of the software. A default setting had to be used instead, which prevented the specific settings used in the verification study to be applied.

The default grid settings led to a grid of 7.6 million cells. Recall that this setup is no longer symmetrical through the centreline, and this would therefore have corresponded to 3.8 million in the verification case (where a grid of 4.3 million cells was preferred). As can be seen in the depiction of the 4 kts case the bare-hull simulations are some ~ 20 % below the test data. Evaluating the results of the verification the following fact can be observed; first, a 20 % error would have been predicted for a grid of only 1.6 million cells, and then for a grid of 3.8 million cells an error of 12.1 % could have been anticipated. This mismatch between results is a consequence of not being able to use the selected grid settings. This also means that the errors of any simulation with the default

Table 3. Comparison of cell densities at different regions. Densities expressed in cells per L_{pp}, y^+ is expressed in dimensionless length unit.

Region (direction)	Verification (*grid* 2)	Investigation
Upstream (longitudinal)	51	140
Bow (longitudinal)	168	280
Midships (longitudinal)	90	127
Transom (longitudinal)	1010	1600
Wake (longitudinal)	101	476
Overall (radial)	42	160
y_1^+	0.7	1.0

grid settings cannot be estimated by the current grid dependence study. The used cell densities are displayed in Table 3.

This means that there are no means of evaluating the error in these simulations. As there is no complete series of heel variation, the trends of these series are not available either, all indicating the need for further research.

5.2   Trim Variation

The results of the trim variation is similar to the heel variation; there are not enough finished simulations to draw any conclusion.

6   Concluding Remarks

6.1   Systematic Variation of Numerical Parameters

This section will sum up the study of systematic variation of numerical parameters. The study included four different parameters that were expected to have an impact on the predicted resistance of the simulations. These simulations were conducted on grids of 4.5 to 6.5 million cells, which turned out to be somewhere at the $\sim 7\,\%$ plateau.

Density Ratio. The result of this study was that the most favorable density ratio was 0.01. The resistance, however, could be increased by 0.90 % by using the physical density ratio, but as this led to very numerically unstable simulations this was not prioritized. The conclusion of this investigation was that the results seem to reach a plateau at 0.005 and the fact that a higher density ratio really did make the simulations more stable. Also, as only a small increase in resistance was observed, it was decided to continue the work with the density ratio set to 0.01.

Domain Height. The domain height had a significant effect on the resistance but also affected the numerical stability of the simulation. Changing the domain height from 0.563 to 0.125 Lpp resulted in a decrease of 2.27 %. Above 0.536 the simulations became too numerically unstable. As the domain height was 0.5 Lpp in the previous simulations already, and the threshold of domain height seemed to be 0.536, the positive effect of increased domain height could not be further exploited. The domain height was therefore kept at 0.5 Lpp.

Concluded from this investigation was that the domain height shall be set to 0.5 Lpp, or in this particular case 2 m, in order to still be in the region of numerical stability but also to give a resistance as close to the towing tank test result as possible.

Turbulence Models. The turbulence models that were implemented for the VOF method in the Shipflow software were EASM and SST $k-\omega$. The previously used SST $k-\omega$ was clearly superior to the EASM in this case. As the EASM predicted a twice-as-large error and took substantially more time to converge, the SST $k-\omega$ was selected.

Cell Density in the Transom Region. The transom region was refined from the previously used 600 cells per Lpp, to 60'000. Only a slight increase in resistance, 0.51 %, was noticed. This study could benefit, however, from more thorough investigation, as it was discovered that cell density in other areas of the hull was greatly affected by the transom area. What can be concluded is that an insufficient resolution in the transom area alone is not a major source of error.

Some of the cases run during the main investigation of this study converged to an oscillating behaviour. This can be due to the fact that the flow is not steady state after all. If the flow is unsteady in the transom region, it can result in that the steady state simulation gives this transom water as a result. To test if the flow is unsteady, a transient simulation has to be done, but as the selected software did not have this option, this was not investigated. Another way of obtaining an unsteady flow in the simulation is if the waves are not small enough when they are leaving the domain. The remedy for this will then be to increase the overall size of the domain in order for the waves to naturally dampen before reaching the boundaries.

6.2 Main Investigation

Though no conclusion can be made regarding where the major source of this $\sim 7\%$ error lies, at least some numerical parameters can be ruled out by this study, facilitating further studies in the area.

The study presented in Sect. 4 took most of the time devoted to this project. As no source for the error was found during this study, the work moved on with a modelling setup that was not accurate. As the objective of this paper is to find a minimum point of a series of heel and trim variations and not necessarily an absolute value, it was still considered possible. The settings selected during this study was to be used in the investigation to the largest possible extent. All grid density settings were not to be kept completely similar, as the investigation would be performed with the boxed grid setup explained in Sect. 2.4.

As explained in Sect. 4.2, keeping similar grid settings was not possible at all. The even-keel bare-hull case was included in the heel and trim variations but resulted in an even lower resistance than during the verification. As there were larger errors than expected by the grid dependence study, the importance of a good grid became even more evident. However, as the error for the verification case increased so dramatically during the investigation, it can also be concluded that the boxed grid does not perform equally well in this case. This conclusion can be made as the verification case was tested with a non-symmetric H-O-grid as well. The resistance was then 6.9 % less than the towing tank test run, compared to the 7.6 % of the symmetric case.

To be able to make decisive conclusions, further investigation needs to be conducted. First of all, decide if the VOF method should be used, and then complete the heel and trim variations. The potential flow method implemented in the software was tested after this study, on the verification case, and predicted the resistance within half a percent.

Here follows a list of suggestions for interesting future research:

Provide Sailing Recommendations. Evaluate the results of the heel and trim variations and make an instruction of how to achieve highest velocity made good, including a VPP study.

Investigate Actual Velocities and Attitudes. Study the sailors to see which velocities and attitudes are common, to see if there is room for improvement.

Tailor for Individual Crew Weights. To really maximize the effect of the individual sailor, a separate investigation for the weight of the individual sailor could be performed.

Acknowledgements. The authors would like to express their gratitude to Professor Lars Larsson, Chalmers University of Technology, Michal Orych, Flowtech International and Matz Brown, SSPA Sweden AB, for their contributions to this paper. Further we acknowledge the financial support provided by Västra Götalandsregionen, Regionutvecklingsnämnden.

References

1. Davidsson, L.: An Introduction to Turbulence Models. Chalmers University of technology, Göteborg (2003)
2. Deng, G.B., Queutey, P., Visonneau, M.: Three dimensional flow computation with reynolds stress and algebraic stress models. In: Engineering Turbulence Modelling and Experiments, vol. 6, pp. 389–398 (2005)
3. Eca, L., Hoekstra, M.: Discretization uncertainty estimation based on a least squaresversion of the grid convergence index. In: 2nd Workshop on CFD Uncertainty Analysis, Lisabon, October 2006
4. Eca, L., Hoekstra, M.: A procedure for the estimation of the numerical uncertainty of CFD calculations based on grid renement studies. J. Comput. Phys. **262**, 104–130 (2014)

5. Feymark, A.: A Large Eddy Simulation Based Fluid-Structure Interaction Methodology with Application in Hydroelasticity. Ph.D. thesis. Chalmers, Göteborg (2013)
6. Gatski, T.B., Speziale, C.G.: On explicit algebraic stress models for complex turbulent fows. J. Fluid Mech. **254**, 59–78 (1993)
7. Hirt, C.W., Nichols, B.-D.: Volume of Fluid (VOF) Method for the Dynamics of Free Boundaries. Los Alamos Scientific Laboratory, New Mexico (1979)
8. Hirt, C.W., Nichols, B.D.: Volume of fluid (VOF) method for the dynamics of free boundaries. J. Comput. Phys. **39**, 201–225 (1998)
9. Larsson, L., Raven, J.: Ship Resistance and Flow. The Society of Naval Architects and Marine Engineers, Jersey City (2010)
10. Marek, M., Aniszewski, W., Boguslawski, A.: Simplified volume of fluid method (SVOF) for two-phase flows. Task Q. **12**(3), 255–265 (2008)
11. Menter, F.R.: Two-equation eddy-viscosity turbulence models for engineering applications. AIAA J. **32**(8), 1598–1605 (1994)
12. Orych, M., Larsson, L., Regnstrom, B.: Adaptive overlapping grid techniques and spatial discretization schemes for increasing surface sharpness and numerical accuracy in free surface capturing methods. In: 28th Symposium on Naval Hydrodynamics, Pasadena California, pp. 389–398 (2010)
13. Roache, P.: Verication and Validation in Computational Science and Engineering. Hermosa Publishers, Socorro (1998)
14. Roy, C.: Grid convergence error analysis for mixed-order numerical schemes. Am. Inst. Aeronaut. Astronaut. **41**, 596–604 (2003)
15. Rumsey, C.: The Menter Shear Stress Transport Turbulence Model. Web Article (2013). http://turbmodels.larc.nasa.gov/sst.html
16. Slater, J.W.: Examining Spatial Grid Convergence. Web Article (2005). http://grc.nasa.gov/WWW/wind/valid/tutorial/
17. Versteeg, H., Malalasekera, W.: An Introduction to Computational Fluid Dynamics: The Finite, vol. Method, 2nd edn. Prentice Hall, Saddle River (2007)
18. Wallin, S., Johansson, A.V.: An explicit algebraic reynolds stress model for incompressible and compressible turbulent flows. Fluid Mech. **403**, 89–132 (2000)
19. Zou, L., Larsson, L.: A verication and validation study based on resistance submissions. In: Larsson, L., Stern, F., Visonneau, M. (eds.) Numerical Ship Hydrodynamics, pp. 203–254. Springer, The Netherland (2010)

Do We Need Goal Line Technology in Soccer or Could Video Proof Be a More Suitable Choice: A Cost-Benefit-Analysis of Goal Line Technology in Soccer and Thoughts About an Introduction of Video Proof

Otto Kolbinger[(✉)], Daniel Linke, Daniel Link, and Martin Lames

Department for Sport and Health Sciences, TU München, Munich, Germany
{otto.kolbinger,daniel.linke,
daniel.link,martin.lames}@tum.de

Abstract. The aim of this study was to investigate the necessity of goal line technology for top level soccer and compare it to video proof. 1167 games of the 1st and 2nd German Bundesliga were screened for critical goal line decisions as well as other critical goal decisions including penalty calls. 16.8 critical goal line decisions were found per season, of which 76.6 % could directly be resolved by tv-review. On average, 5.0 and 2.8 cases were found respectively in the 1st and 2nd Bundesliga that could justify goal line technology. Furthermore, just 5.0 % of all critical calls concerned goal-line decisions, while 84.3 % involve offside, representing the main reason for critical goal calls. Based on these findings, in terms of a cost-benefit-relation, a video proof could be more suitable than goal line technology. Consequently, we discuss the obstacles and preconditions for the introduction of a video proof in soccer.

Keywords: Goal line technology · Video proof · Soccer

1 Introduction

For scoring a goal in Soccer the whole of the ball has to pass the goal line, according to the official laws of the game [1] of the Fédération Internationale de Football Association (FIFA). History shows that this easy fact could be arguable in seldom cases. Perhaps the oldest instance was the fifth goal of the 1966 World Cup final between England and Germany. With the game tied in extra time, a shot of the English striker Geoff Hurst hit the underside of the crossbar, bounced down towards the line and hit the ground near the goal line. The referee and his linesman respectively decided that the ball had passed the goal line completely. Whether this call was right (or wrong) was solved only 1996, when a study of Reid and Zisserman [2] concluded that the ball didn't cross the line entirely by at least six centimeters. In Germany, this famous incident led to the expression "Wembley Goal" for disputed goal calls, after the ball hitting the underside of the crossbar.

© Springer International Publishing Switzerland 2015
J. Cabri et al. (Eds.): icSPORTS 2014, CCIS 556, pp. 107–118, 2015.
DOI: 10.1007/978-3-319-25249-0_8

In recent years technologies became available which are able to track the position of the ball and therefore can decide if the ball crossed the goal line. Thus, the International Football Association Board (IFAB) decided to permit goal line technology in July 2012. To get accredited as FIFA licensed goal line technology providers, a company has to pass a series of certain tests, including laboratory tests as well as field tests [3]. The two main requirements are an accuracy of 1.5 cm (3.0 cm before 2014) and the indication of whether a goal has been scored must be communicated to the referee in less than one second.

So far, the FIFA has officially accredited four systems, representing two different technologies. The camera based systems use several high speed cameras which are located around the pitch, continuously capturing the ball's position in three dimensions when it is close to the goal. The Hawk-Eye system is already used e.g. in the English Premier League, GoalControl was the official provider for the 2014 FIFA World Cup[TM]. For these systems no modifications or adaptions of the ball are necessary. Magnetic-field-based systems need the implication of receptors in the ball, for enabling the system to calculate the position of the ball. The accredited systems using this technology were run by the Frauenhofer Institute for Integrated Circuits and by ChyronHego.

The study was commissioned and funded by Deutsche Fußball Liga (DFL, trans. German Football League) [5] in the run up of a general meeting on March 24th 2014. On a vote at this meeting, delegates of the clubs of German 1st and 2nd Bundesliga decided to not introduce goal line technology in these two leagues. The discussion about the introduction of a goal line technology didn't stop in the aftermath of this meeting. Thus, in a second vote, at the general meeting on December 4th 2014, the delegates approved the use of goal line technology at least in the 1st Bundesliga.

Scientific research concerning GLT so far mostly centers on technological issues [4]. Up to now, there is no study investigating in how far the implementation of this new technology is necessary in terms of a cost-benefit-relation. For example the costs for the installation and maintenances of Hawk-Eye systems can be set for round about 2.30 million euro per season (for a league with 18 stadiums). Therefore this study examines the frequency of critical goal-line situations in order to put these costs in perspective with these frequency. In addition, it was obtained how many of these critical incidents could be solved with videos provided by the usual TV-footage. Since the very majority of professional soccer matches is recorded by several cameras, this method should illustrate a procedure of checking critical goal-line decisions without (or just with low) extra expenses.

The method of scoring, according to the official laws of the game, also requires "that no infringement of the Laws of the Game has been committed previously by the team scoring the goal" [1]. So the number of critical goal-line situations was compared to other sources of disputed decisions, i.e. offside, handling the ball, foul and penalty calls. These situations were also checked with the TV-footage. So far, the IFAB didn't approve any kind of video replay. The concerns of changing the nature of the game outweigh the possible advantages, but the topic shall still be discussed at the IFAB's Annual General Meetings. Thus, this study also investigated the necessity and enlightenment rate of a video replay.

Due to the nature of soccer there are also other issues concerning the introduction of new technologies. The use of video proof would need rules for the video proof itself as well as its embedding in the current laws of the game. Based on sports that already use video proof we discuss its possible regulations and the necessary (rule) preconditions for its introduction in soccer.

2 Methods

2.1 Database

The sample contained matches from day 18 of the 2011/2012 season to day 20 of the 2013/2014 season of 1st and 2nd German Bundesliga. The DFL provided footage of 1167 of these matches via their database Deutsches Fußball Archiv. Even since this footage is rather an offer for the media than for performance analysis or scientific researches, it included all available camera angles as well as slow-motion replays. The number of available camera angles varied from seven (e.g. low priority 2nd Bundesliga matchup) to 22 cameras (e.g. nationwide broadcasted matches). The results section will include numbers per match day (or round) and per season which were extrapolated based on the sample of the 1167 matches.

2.2 Operationalization

Critical Goal Line Decisions. It was assumed that the frequency of goal line technology uses would be determined by the frequency of scenes that arouse the suspicion that a goal line decision could be critical. This includes situations were a goal was called as well as when the referee decided that the ball didn't crossed the goal line. This led to the following two definitions:

1. A goal is called, but the ball doesn't touch the net
2. The ball approaches the goal line by less than one diameter, before or after it gets deflected, with players of the offensive team complaining because of the goal-line decision

The second definition includes a positional precondition as well as a certain behavior of the offensive players. There are several scenes in a soccer match with the ball approaching the goal line by less than one diameter but it is obvious for all the involved people that no goal was scored. So the second definition includes protests of players of the offensive team.

Critical Goal Decisions. To quantify the rate of critical goal line decisions of all critical goal calls, critical goals due to other sources were obtained. A goal was called critical by fulfilling at least one of the following three rule infringements by the scoring team:

- Offside: Involved player (of the offensive team) is offside in a certain period of time, from 0.25 s before until 0.25 s after the last touch of a teammate
- Foul: Defensive player loses body control due to a contact with an involved offensive player
- Handling the ball: Involved offensive player touches the ball with his hand, arm or shoulder

Besides these kinds of critical goals all penalties were captured.

2.3   Video Replay

All critical goal line decisions as well as critical calls were evaluated and double-checked by two experts using the provided TV-footage. After the review the call was rated as "correct", "false" or "not to decide clearly". When a critical goal line decision was "not to decide clearly" by video replay, it was concluded that this scene could only be solved by using goal line technology. Penalty calls were just rated as "doubtless" or "doubtful", due to influences like the interpretation of the laws of the game by the referee. Thereby "doubtless" included just scenes in which the referee's call was obviously right, assuming that the other calls could arouse suspicion that the penalty call was disputable. Due to the nature of this study, as it was commissioned by the DFL, all these evaluations had to be double-checked by both experts.

2.4   Reliability

The reliability of the observation method was investigated with an inter-rater reliability study. Therefore the matches of three randomly selected game days (i.e. 27 matches) were investigated independently by both experts. The reliability was measured using Cohen's Kappa for the identification of critical goals and the source of critical goal decisions. As mentioned above, it wasn't possible to check the inter-rater-agreement of the evaluations, since the evaluations had to be double-checked anyway. Both variables showed a very good strength of agreement (according to the suggested limits of Altmann [5]), with k-values of 0.95 and 1.0 for the identification and the source respectively. Even by suggesting more strict limits for easier variables, or almost obvious variables like the source of critical goal decisions, the classification of the inter-rater-agreement can be kept up.

3   Results

3.1   Critical Goal Line Decisions

For the investigated 613 matches of the 1st German Bundesliga 39 scenes were identified that arouse the suspicion that a goal line decision could be critical. As shown in Table 1, that means that per game day 0.58 and per season 19.6 critical goal line decisions appear. In the 2nd German Bundesliga these rates were lower. 25 critical goal line decisions were found in 554 matches, meaning 0.41 per round and 13.9 per season.

Table 1. Scenes in which goal line technology would be mandatory and critical goal line decisions (in brackets) of the German Bundesliga and 2nd Bundesliga.

	Bundesliga		2nd Bundesliga	
total	10	(39)	5	(25)
per match	0.02	(0.06)	0.01	(0.05)
per round	0.15	(0.58)	0.08	(0.41)
per season	5.02	(19.6)	2.78	(13.9)

As mentioned above, critical goal line decisions which were rated as "not to decide clearly" by video reviews were classified as scenes that could only have been solved by goal line technology. For the 1st German Bundesliga 5.02 such scenes were found per seasons, meaning 0.15 per round and 0.02 per match. For the 2nd German Bundesliga these numbers are lower, too. 2.78 scenes per season had been identified, meaning 0.08 per game day and 0.01 per match. Regarding the detection rate of critical goal line decisions by video proof, the results showed that 76.6 % of these situations could be solved with the available TV-footage.

3.2   Critical Goal Decisions

Prevalence. The rates of critical goals are listed in Table 2. The table includes critical goals due to critical goal line calls as well as possible infringements of the law of the game by the offensive team. The results show that 4.72 % and 5.59 % of all critical goals were critical because of goal line calls in the 1st and 2nd Bundesliga respectively. Offside calls were the major source for critical goal decisions, with 85.0 % in the 1st Bundesliga and 83.2 % in the 2nd Bundesliga. Foul (5.91 %) and handling the ball (4.33 %) are in the same range as critical goal line decisions in the 1st Bundesliga. In the 2nd Bundesliga of the 554 screened matches of this league, critical goals due to possible fouls (9.79 %) have a slightly bigger rate, while only two goals in total were critical due to handling.

Table 2. Critical goal decisions in the 1st and 2nd Bundesliga by source of doubt and their rate of all the critical goals per league in percent (in brackets).

	Offside	Handling	Foul	Goal line
1st Bundesliga	216	11	15	12
	(85.0)	(4.33)	(5.91)	(4.72)
2nd Bundesliga	119	2	14	8
	(83.2)	(1.40)	(9.79)	(5.59)

Penalties. In total 310 penalties were called in the investigated 1167 matches, or rather 0.27 per game in the 1st Bundesliga and 0.26 per game in the 2nd Bundesliga. Fouls were a more frequent rule infringement leading to penalties with 81.7 % (1st Bundesliga) and 83.6 % (2nd Bundesliga).

20.6 % of all penalty calls (foul: 19.6 %, handling: 25.9 %) were rated as "doubtful" by TV-review and therefore as critical goal calls. Regarding the success rates of 81.7 % (1st Bundesliga) and 74.0 % (2nd Bundesliga), this means that there were 0.39 critical goals per round due to their preceding penalty calls.

Video Replay. After thorough video inspections, all critical goal calls were rated as "correct", "false" or "not to decide clearly". As mentioned above, the detection rate for critical goal line decisions is 76.6 %. Figure 1 illustrates the detection rates for all sources of critical goals as well as the rate of all investigated critical decisions. The highest values were reached for offside decisions with 89.3 % and fouls with 86.2 %. The lowest detection rate showed handling calls (86.2 %). In total 86.6 % of all the investigated critical calls could be solved with video-replays based on the available TV-footage.

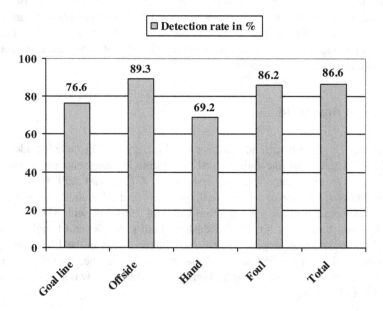

Fig. 1. Detection rate of critical goal line calls (also including scenes were no goal was called) and critical goal calls sorted by category and in total.

4 Discussion

4.1 Prevalence of Critical Goal Line Decisions and Other Critical Goal Calls

The results of this investigation show that merely 5.0 % of all critical goal decisions concern the question whether the ball completely passed the goal line or not. Furthermore, the frequency of these decisions is very low with 0.02 per match in the 1st German Bundesliga and 0.01 in the 2nd Bundesliga respectively. This means, using Bernoulli distributions, that per stadium per season in the 1st Bundesliga the probability of having at least one case were the use of goal line technology would be non-negotiable is just 0.24. This probability is even lower in the 2nd Bundesliga (0.14). Figure 2 also shows that these probabilities are over 95 % only after eleven full seasons in the 1st Bundesliga and 20 seasons in the 2nd Bundesliga. Regarding the 135.00 € per stadium per season, there is a potential chance of spending this money without getting any kind of benefit.

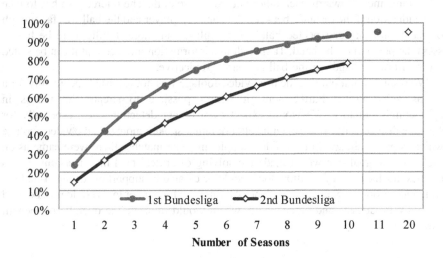

Fig. 2. Bernoulli probabilities for at least one non-negotiable use of goal line technology in one stadium for 1st and 2nd Bundesliga from one to ten seasons and (after the vertical line) the number of seasons until this probability reaches 95 %

Other sources for critical goal calls outnumber critical goal calls by far. Especially offside, which represents the major reason for disputable goal decisions with approximately 85 %. In the 1st Bundesliga appeared one critical goal – excluding critical goal line decisions – at least every three games (0.39 per game), and in the 2nd Bundesliga almost in one game out of four. These numbers exclude critical goals because of disputable penalty calls, which adds another 0.39 such goals per round.

All these critical goal calls couldn't be solved with goal line technology. Video proof could be a possible solution to solve them. Since every match in the two German Bundesligen is recorded by at least seven (up to 22) cameras this technology would have a much better cost-benefit-relation. And this technology could solve such calls as well as critical goal line decisions.

4.2   Rate of Enlightenment

86.6 % of all the investigated critical calls could be clearly solved with the provided TV-footage, including the solved 76.6 % of critical goal lines decisions. The highest detection rate was reached for critical offside decisions (89.3 %), followed by disputable foul calls and no-calls respectively (86.2 %). The rate of enlightenment for handling the ball was the lowest with 69.2 %. This could be a consequence of the rule, which interpretation is partly subjective based on vague definitions in the official laws of the game [1]. For example, the referee has to decide whether the ball moves towards the hand or the hand moves towards the ball. Usually both move and due to the nature of the game move towards each other not exactly seldom. The referee also has to take in consideration if the distance between the handling player and the ball was far enough so that it isn't an "unexpected ball" for the player anymore. Furthermore he has to assess the position of the hand. Taking all this information into account it can be stated that the rules for handling the ball are partly subjective.

We want to point out that the used video-footage was not recorded specifically for a use as video proof. Furthermore, it wasn't possible to stream the videos in high-definition-quality. We would expect even higher detection rates, especially for objective decisions like offside, with better or rather spoken more specific video-footage (which is partly already in use). For example, in some matches there were cameras on level with the goal line which made the solving of critical goal line decisions in this matches much easier. In addition, tools could be created to support the decision-making with video-proofs, e.g. an offside-plane. All this new footage or tools could also be used in the TV-broadcasts and other media, which would improve the overall cost-benefit ratio.

4.3   Obstacles and Pre-considerations for the Introduction
of Video-Replay

Obstacles. There are generally two main objections to the introduction of a video proof in soccer. One is the nostalgic point of view, that disputable calls are a part of the game and could be a reason for the popularity of soccer. Of course, there are instances of games that were especially famous because of critical goal calls, e.g. the above-mentioned World Cup final of 1966. But the introduction of goal line technology shows that this traditional mindset is already given up by the FIFA and the IFAB.

The other main doubt is the change of the nature of the game. It is supposed that the introduction of a video replay would lead to more and/or longer interruptions of the game. For verifying this thesis two different topics have to be taken into account:

the possible duration of a video replay and the already given pattern of interruptions in soccer matches. On average there are well over 100 interruptions in elite men soccer matches and the total duration of all interruptions is 30 to 40 min, meaning approximately a third of the compete match time [7, 8]. The interruptions after goals and before penalties are on average already over 50 s, which could be enough for video replays. Free kicks merely take twenty seconds but last significant longer in the offensive areas of the pitch [8].

A current pilot scheme of the Koninklijke Nederlandse Voetbal Bond (KNVB, tans. Royal Dutch Soccer Association) suggests that video replay interventions should last 15 s at maximum [9]. But this project focuses only on the avoidance of obvious mistakes and there are no results published yet. However, there are no empirical values showing how long video replays could last in soccer. Consequently, the experiences of other sports, that already use video proof, should be taken as reference. The Major League Baseball expanded their replay rules in beginning of the 2014 season, so for example tag plays and force plays became reviewable [10]. As different as soccer and baseball are, replays of these two types of call could deliver valuable hints for the duration of replays in soccer. Both types of decisions are based on very objective rules. For critical force play calls the referee has to check whether the runner touches the base before the defensive player (touching the same base) catches the ball or not. For tag plays it has to be verified if the runner was touched with the ball (or the glove that holds the ball).

The official time data of all such 823 replays from 1st of May 2014 until the end of the regular season 2014 were investigated. The information used here was obtained free of charge from and is copyrighted by Retrosheet [10]. The average duration was 01:43 min with the median at 01:35. As shown in Fig. 3, none of the replays was

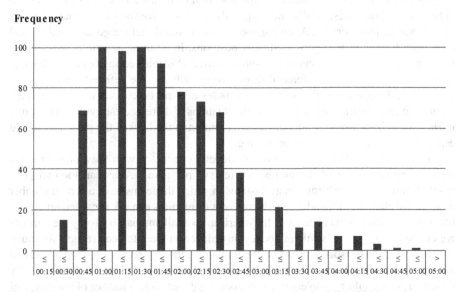

Fig. 3. Frequencies of the durations of force and tag plays in the MLB 2014 regular season, excluding games in April. The range of values are set as 15 s.

shorter than 15 s and only 1.82 % were shorter than 30 s. Half of the replays (from percentile rank 25 to 75) lastet between 1:04 and 02:14, while there were also durations of up to 4:46 detected.

Even considering the different circumstances in baseball, where the time of interruptions isn't a factor (yet), the set 15 s of the KNVB seem to be unrealistic. On the other hand, regarding the average durations of interruptions for goals and penalties, it at least doesn't seem impossible to evaluate the specific calls during the period of these interruptions.

Pre-considerations. For an introduction of video replays new regulations for its use would be necessary. Starting with the consideration, based on the thoughts above, which calls should be reviewable and when. In this context, "when" means in which state of the game. When the referee evaluates a critical situation he just interrupts the game if he decides that there was an infringement of the laws of the game (or the ball passed the goal line for critical goal line decisions). In this case a replay could be used without large-scale rule changes, but how could calls be reviewed where the referee doesn't interrupt the game? This question does not occur in sports that are interrupted after every play like baseball or American football. Hockey is also an invasion game (like soccer) and already uses video replays. Unfortunately, this problem isn't satisfyingly solved in the official hockey regulations [12]. It is determined that the referee can stop the game, but not the restart-scenario for video replays that result in no-calls, i.e. situations in which the game wouldn't be interrupted. Possibilities could be a drop ball or a free kick for the team that was in possession before the game was interrupted for the replay. The main problem will be to re-establish a game situation, when one team had an advantage at the moment of the interruption, at worst some kind of scoring opportunity.

This problem could be avoided by the selection of reviewable calls. In Hockey the video umpire should especially (but explicitly not exclusive) assist for goals, penalty strokes and penalty corners. A similar use in soccer would include goals, penalties and eventually free kicks in highly promising positions. In all these situations there would be interruptions of decent intervals as shown above. Possible scoring opportunities that were taken away by the referee due to wrong calls by the referee would remain unresolved. To overcome this source of disputes it could be conceivable encouraging referees to just interrupt the game in such situations if there is clear evidence of a rule infringement. This would be an indirect intervention in the laws of the game and would especially change the nature of refereeing.

Another fact that has to be considered, directly connected with the aforementioned facts, is the regulation of the number of replays per game. American football [13], baseball and hockey each run replay systems in which the teams have a certain number of so-called challenges. In addition, the referees or umpires can ask for video replays as often as (they think it is) necessary. In American football and baseball only the coaches are entitled to challenge, while in hockey any player on the pitch can request for video proof. A good fit for soccer could be the implementation of parts of the replay system in American football. In so called booth-reviews all scoring plays are automatically reviewed. This could be implemented for soccer without direct changes of the nature of the game, even by including penalty calls. Of course, this could still lead to indirect changes, for example due to adapted refereeing styles.

Furthermore, there are different possibilities for the process of video replays. In the MLB umpires in the league's headquarter evaluate the calls and give the requesting umpires feedback. In hockey the referees refer decisions to video umpires that sit in a kind of broadcast unit in the direct proximity of the pitch or stadium respectively. The project of the KNVB works with this process. It might also be conceivable to give the forth official the task of doing the video replays.

5 Conclusion

The results of this study show that there are several disputable calls in soccer matches and previous studies proofed that limits of the human perception are a reason for it. As one source of error, for example, the flash-lag effect was identified uniformly [14, 15] while another source is still controversially discussed (optical error hypothesis) [16–18]. The IFAB and the FIFA already accommodated this issue and approved the use of goal line technologies. The results of this study showed that this technology has a disputable cost-benefit-relation as only 5.0 % of all critical goals concern goal line decisions.

The Introduction of a video proof seems to be a more suitable choice as 86.6 % of all critical goal calls, including critical goal line decisions, could be resolved by using only the usual TV-footage. Based on knowledge about interruptions in soccer and experiences with video proofs in other sports, we could show that the inclusion of a video replay could be possible without large-scaled changes of the nature of the game. The introduction of a booth-review, as in American football, reviewing all scoring plays and penalty calls, might be promising.

References

1. Fédération Internationale de Football Association. http://www.fifa.com/mm/document/footballdevelopment/refereeing/81/42/36/log2013en_neutral.pdf
2. Reid, I., Zisserman, A.: Goal-directed video metrology. In: Cipolla, R., Buxton, B. (eds.) Computer Vision – ECCV'96. LNCS, vol. 2, pp. 647–658. Springer, Heidelberg (1996)
3. Fédération Internationale de Football Association. http://www.fifa.com/mm/document/affederation/administration/02/35/96/73/fifa-background-paper_glt_june2014_en_neutral.pdf
4. Spagnolo, P., Leo, M., Mazzeo, P.L., Nitti, M., Stella, E., Distante, A.: Non-Invasive soccer goal line technology: a real case study. In: 2013 IEEE Conference on Computer Vision and Pattern Recognition Workshops, pp. 1011–1018. Conference Publishing Services, Los Alamitos (2013)
5. Kolbinger, O., Linke, D., Link, D., Lames, M.: Zur Notwendigkeit von Torlinientechnologie in den Fußball-Bundesligen. Deutsche Fußball Liga GmbH, Frankfurt (2014)
6. Altmann, D.G.: Practical Statistics for Medical Research. Chapman and Hall, London (1991)

7. Augste, C., Lames, M.: Differenzierte betrachtung von taktischem verhalten und belastungsstrukturen auf der basis von spielunterbrechungen im fussball. In: Woll, A., Klöckner, W., Reichmann, M., Schlag, M. (eds.), Sportspielkulturen erfolgreich gestalten, pp. 113–116. Czwalina, Hamburg (2008)
8. Siegle, M., Lames, M.: Game interruptions in elite soccer. J. Sports Sci. **30**(7), 619–624 (2012)
9. Koninklijke Nederlandse Voetbal Bond. http://english.knvb.nl/content/485/refereeing-20
10. Major League Baseball. http://mlb.mlb.com/mlb/official_info/official_rules/replay_review. jsp
11. Retrosheet. http://www.retrosheet.org/replays.htm
12. International Hockey Federation. http://www.fieldhockey.ca/files/Officials%20Resources/ FIH%20Tournament%20Regulations%20Outdoor%20-%20January%202013.pdf
13. National Football League. https://www.nfl.info/download/2012mediaguides/%20nfl%20rule %20book.pdf
14. Gillis, B., Helsen, W., Catteeuw, P., Van Roie, E., Wagemans, J.: Interpretation and application of the offside law by expert assistant referees: perception of spatial positions in complex dynamic events on and off the field. J. Sports Sci. **27**(6), 551–563 (2009)
15. Helsen, W., Gillis, B., Weston, M.: Errors in judging "offside" in football: test oft he optical error versus the perceptual flash-lag hypothesis. J. Sports Sci. **24**(5), 521–528 (2006)
16. Oudejans, R.R.D., Verheijen, R., Bakker, F.C., Gerrits, J.C., Steinbrückner, M., Beek, P.J.: Errors in judging "offside" in football. Nature **404**, 33 (2000)
17. Oudejans, R.R.D., Bakker, F.C., Beek, P.J.: Helsen, gillis and weston (2006) err in testing the optical error hypothesis. J. Sport Sci. **25**(9), 987–990 (2007)
18. Helsen, W., Gillis, B., Weston, M.: Helsen, gillis and weston (2006) do not err in questioning the optical error hypothesis as the only major account for explaining offside decision-making errors. J. Sport Sci. **25**(9), 991–994 (2007)

Author Index

Printed in the United States
By Bookmasters